S0-BOW-710

Personnel Administration in the Health Services Industry

Health Systems Management
Edited by **Samuel Levey, Ph.D.,** *University of Iowa*

Volume 1:
Financial Management of Health Institutions
J.B. Silvers and C.K. Prahalad
ISBN 0-470-79173-X 1974

Volume 2:
Personnel Administration in the Health Services Industry: Theory & Practice
Norman Metzger
ISBN 0-470-59993-6 1974

Volume 3:
The National Labor Relations Act: A Guidebook for Health Care Facility Administrators
Dennis D. Pointer and Norman Metzger
ISBN 0-470-69146-8 1975

Volume 4:
Organizational Issues in Health Care Management
Alan Sheldon
ISBN 0-470-78275-7 1975

Volume 5:
Long Term Care: A Handbook for Researchers, Planners and Providers
Sylvia Sherwood, Editor
ISBN 0-470-78600-0 1975

Volume 6:
Analysis of Urban Health Problems: Case Studies from the Health Services Administration
of the City of New York
Irving Leveson and Jeffrey H. Weiss, Editors
ISBN 0-470-14983-3 1976

Volume 7:
Health Maintenance Organizations: A Guide to Planning and Development
Roger W. Birnbaum
ISBN 0-470-14984-1 1976

Volume 8:
Labor Arbitration in Health Care
Earl R. Baderschneider and Paul F. Miller, Editors
ISBN 0-470-15037-8 1976

Volume 9:
The Consumer and the Health Care System: Social and Managerial Perspectives
Harry Rosen, Jonathan M. Metsch and Samuel Levey, Editors
ISBN 0-89335-005-2 1977

Volume 10:
Long-Term Care Administration: A Managerial Perspective, I & II
Samuel Levey and N. Paul Loomba, Editors
ISBN 0-89335-004-4 (I) 1977
ISBN 0-89335-015-X (II) 1977

Volume 11:
Hospital Organization and Management: Text and Readings, 2nd Ed.
Jonathon S. Rakich and Kurt Darr, Editors
ISBN 0-89335-029-X 1978

Volume 12:
Democratic Processes for Modern Health Agencies
Irving Ladimer with Joel C. Solomon and Stanley G. House
ISBN 0-89335-042-7 1979

362.10683
m568p

Personnel Administration in the Health Services Industry

Second Edition

Norman Metzger

Vice President for Personnel,
Mount Sinai Medical Center, New York

WITHDRAWN

SP

SP MEDICAL & SCIENTIFIC BOOKS

a division of Spectrum Publications, Inc.
New York • London

LIBRARY ST. MARY'S COLLEGE
161093

To my grandchildren—Tiel, Brooke and Erica

Copyright © 1979 Spectrum Publications, Inc.

All rights reserved. No part of this book may be reproduced in any form, by photostat, microfilm, retrieval system, or any other means without prior written permission of the copyright holder or his licensee,

SPECTRUM PUBLICATIONS, INC.
175-20 Wexford Terrace, Jamaica, N.Y. 11432

Library of Congress Cataloging in Publication Data

Metzger, Norman, 1924-
    Personnel administration in the health services industry.

    Includes index.
    1. Health facilities—Personnel management.
    2. Collective bargaining—Health facilities.
    I. Title.
    RA971.35.M474 1979   658.3'7'3621   78-31330
    ISBN 0-89335-074-5

Fourth Printing, April 1984

PREFACE

The primary aim of hospitals and homes is the rendering of the highest quality of patient care. Often overlooked yet nevertheless true, efficient patient care develops not from the quality of medical knowledge alone nor from modern medical equipment and drugs alone, but from a combination of all those things *and* a well-motivated, well-administered and well-rewarded work force. When one talks about the health care industry, one is addressing himself to the most complex and diversified grouping of employees in any industry. The assemblage of people—professionals, para-professionals, skilled and nonskilled—in an efficient group fully cognizant of institutional goals and committed to their fulfillment is not happenstance. It is carefully planned with maximum input and participation by all parties and the result of professional administration. The road to perdition is strewn with cadavers of administrators of hospitals and homes who pontificated upon their uniqueness rather than *tooling up* for the complex responsibility of delivering quality patient care at acceptable levels of cost. *Tooling up* includes the commitment to and design of programs for the maximizing of employee and institutional contribution to current social and individual goals. *This can only be realized as health care administrators accept personnel administration as one of their more important responsibilities.*

The institutional milieu and its methods of operation in general must be so arranged that employees from doctors to porters can achieve their goals by directing their efforts toward the institutional objectives. Achieving individual goals and institutional objectives are not mutually exclusive. A proficient personnel department led by a professional personnel director can add immeasurably to the fabric of the institution as it pertains to the delivery of sound and quality patient care.

The last paragraph of this book quotes Dale Yoder:

> Manpower management must give more attention to the satisfaction of fundamental, psychological and social needs of employees if it is to perform its function with greatest effectiveness.[1]

The highly sophisticated and complex environments now operative in hospitals and homes cry out for the appointment and development of competent and thinking individuals as personnel directors in those institutions. In the last chapter, I list 14 of the most important responsibilities of the personnel director. In order to fulfill these responsibilities and translate that action into the improvement of the lot of people at work and the realization of institutional goals, the theory and practice of sound personnel administration is essential.

The need to codify the principles and policies of personnel administration in health care facilities is clear and present. I have translated this into a book which was written to provide something more than the philosophy and underlying principles of manpower management in hospitals and homes: a handbook which directs the reader's attention to not only the "why" but the "how" of personnel programs. Throughout each of the chapters of this book the reader will be exposed to both theory and practice. Forms are liberally exhibited. When the various positions in a personnel department are discussed, job descriptions of those positions are presented. In the discussion of job analysis, a job information form is exhibited. The practitioner in the field—personnel administrators at all levels—and administrators of hospitals and homes will find this book more a handbook on "how to" than a theoretical exposition.

It is difficult to translate into appropriate recognition the unselfish assistance of Marlin "Bud" Cruse in getting out the final manuscript. He did more than type and edit, though that was a prodigious effort in itself. He suggested, insisted on and convinced me to make numerous changes which, I believe, have benefited the final product; he reviewed each chapter; he directed my attention to clarify, amplify and modify, where necessary. This is his book as well as mine.

I am indebted to the following people who have permitted me to adapt material that they have developed and to incorporate their labors into this book: Dr. Leslie M. Slote, Dr. Neil Miller, George Kaufman, Arthur Pell, Norman Hirsch and all the members of the Personnel Department of The Mount Sinai Medical Center. I would like to acknowledge those organizations that have granted me the permission to reprint previously published materials: The American Management Association, New York, N.Y.; The Conference Board, New York, N.Y.; Hospital Research and Education Trust, Chicago, Ill.: Training Research and Special Studies Division of the United Hospital Fund, New York, N.Y.; Industrial Relations Counselors Service, New York, N.Y.; Miller-Ginsberg Associates, LaFayette Hill, Pa.; American Society for Hospital Personnel Administration, Chicago, Ill.; and

The Association of Hospital Personnel Administrators of Greater New York, New York, N.Y.

This book is the product of the many authors cited in the text, of the people and institutions acknowledged above and of my long years—too long to admit—of experience in industrial personnel administration and health care personnel administration.

In addition, it brings together all the research I have done in over 20 years of teaching at Bernard M. Baruch College of The City University of New York; Columbia University; Teachers College of Columbia; The New School for Social Research; and The New York State School of Industrial and Labor Relations Extension Program, Cornell University.

In the final analysis, it is a labor of love.

Norman Metzger
New York, New York

Notes

1. Dale Yoder, *Personnel Principles and Practices* (Englewood Cliffs, N.J.: Prentice Hall, 1956), p. 9.

CONTENTS

Chapter

Personnel Administration
in the Health Services Industry

I. HISTORICAL DEVELOPMENT OF MANPOWER MANAGEMENT

Personnel administration is a relatively new discipline within the health services industry. Although modern personnel administration developed at the turn of the century on the industrial scene, it was not until mid-century that hospitals, homes and other health care facilities addressed their attention to the professional management of the personnel function.

The Profession of Personnel Management

The function of providing manpower resources and effective leadership in their utilization in the interest of developing a highly motivated and smooth-running work force is performed by all supervisors, managers and executives of an organization, but it is institutionalized in the personnel department. In organizations that are large enough to warrant it, personnel practitioners are employed in a separate staff unit or department. Therefore, the growth of personnel occupations parallels in general the development and growth of the modern organization and, specifically, the development and growth of the personnel department and its function within organizations.[1]

Personnel management, though a comparatively new art in the health services industry, is based upon such old and well-established disciplines as economics, psychology, anthropology, sociology and even political science. The field of psychology has provided the personnel manager with information that has been applied to employee training, testing, selection and placement, and to an essential part of the delivery of quality patient care: motivation. It is difficult to think of fruitful labor relations and wage and salary administration without a background in economics. Anthropology has served to show how individuals react to the organizational environment and the social system which they join; it has provided insight into the attitudes and, indeed, the myths that people bring to the job. The under-

1

standing of group activities and the effects upon employees of group membership and communications filters down to the personnel administrator from the field of sociology. The understanding of organization and authority relationships emanates from the political science arena.[2]

Welfarism and Scientific Management

Managements in their desire to improve the general standard of living of the American worker introduced certain facilities and programs to neutralize the generally imposed, arduous working conditions which they had experienced. This *welfarism,* or *paternalism,* produced recreational programs, financial assistance for education and medical care, and improved hygienic measures in the working milieu. With the passage of Workmen's Compensation laws, employers not in the least altruistic instituted programs designed to reduce and prevent work injuries and to organize company health programs.[3] New positions developed as a result of welfarism and scientific management, e.g., those of safety engineer, safety director, company physician, industrial nurse and medical director.

The greatest impetus toward the development of a centralized personnel function came from Frederick W. Taylor. Taylor's theories incorporated a fundamental precept that selection, placement and training of workers could no longer be undertaken in a haphazard, rule-of-thumb manner, but must be conducted on a systematic, procedural basis with a high degree of specialization. It is true that the first personnel departments were manned by the "hail-fellow well met" type who saw their position as primarily one of buying loyalty, curbing unionism and engendering a happy spirit in the fashion of Y.M.C.A. directors. While at the turn of the century industrial firms employed social or welfare secretaries, the true beginnings of modern personnel administration can be traced to The National Cash Register Company. In 1902 this firm introduced a labor department to deal with workmen's grievances and unjust labor practices. Close on the heels of this new experiment in employer relations was the inauguration of an employment department in 1910 at Blimpton Press whose original responsibility was hiring and record-keeping, which soon developed to include the area of savings in the *human cost of industry.* Eilbert points out that Dartmouth College at its Tuck School offered the first training program for employment managers in 1915.[4] It is interesting to note that the first personnel departments were really employment sections. It is not difficult to understand that this same development occurred in the health services industry. For the first half of the twentieth century, the personnel function in the health care industry was as an employment service. A senior clerical person was delegated the responsibility of screening applicants, running ads and keeping records. None could do more; none were permitted to do more.

The Roots of Modern Personnel Administration

The earliest work relationships were based upon the principle of slavery. Masters owned and commanded as many workers as they could support. There was very little attention to waste since slaves were available if one could feed them. The slave owners assumed many of the functions that one associates with modern personnel administration, e.g., recruitment (the cruel but efficient method of enslaving and transporting able-bodied men), training, housing, catering and industrial medicine. *The one discipline that was conspicuously absent was collective bargaining.*

During the Middle Ages the serf system was highly developed. Serfs, in contrast to the slaves, enjoyed certain privileges since they were not chattels but were attached to the land which they worked. Such a system could only exist in an agricultural society. The handicraft system, which was the true forerunner of the modern industrial society, encompassed craftsmen who worked in their own homes and hired others. Such craftsmen took younger men, apprentices, and taught them the trade. Apprentices were paid little, if anything, and lived with their masters. Once they reached the journeyman's status, they could move from one craftsman to another, and if they could save money and purchase a few tools they could start their own business. From this system craft guilds developed. These were associations which regulated the quality of materials, wages paid and terms and conditions of apprenticeship training. In the handicraft system personnel management was the responsibility of the master craftsman. Such a system existed only where there was no permanent class of wage earners. Again, collective bargaining was conspicuous by its absence. The industrial revolution changed all that had preceded. With the expansion of markets, better transportation, the development of machines which replaced hand tools and steam power, the workers' efforts could be multiplied. This also produced a requirement for greater capital. New social and economic classes emerged. Wage earners for the first time formed a distinct class. Industrial capitalists provided the money for larger, more complex enterprises. Slowly, but perceptibly, a changing attitude toward the worker developed. There was a growing emphasis on personal and individual values. Workers could move to areas where free land was available, and for the first time employers realized a dissatisfied employee could generally become an independent landowner or farmer.

Personnel management went through dramatic changes. Paternalistic at first, it was then shaped to prevent or undermine unions; finally, it evolved into a professional approach to the managing of manpower. This last period saw personnel management being delegated to a professional group of thoroughly trained specialists.

Functions of the Personnel Department

"Hospitals are people."[5]

Labor and labor-associated expenses make up more than 70 percent of the average hospital's total budget. Nowhere can one find a more complex organization than the modern hospital. Although the complexity of such organizations varies with size, the functions normally delegated to the personnel department are universal. Pigors and Myers list the range of problems which confront a personnel department:

1. Recruitment, selection and placement—centralized hiring procedures; subsidiary policy requirements; requisitioning workers; recruitment and sources of labor supplies; selection through the employment interview, the application blank, the physical examination and employment tests; placement on the right job.

2. Selection and training of supervisors—the supervisor's functions and responsibilities; methods of selecting supervisors; training for future supervisors; specific training for present supervisors.

3. Employee induction and training—responsibility for induction and training; induction as a part of training; types of employee training; developing a training program; training techniques; training as a continuing function.

4. Employee rating and promotion—what a good rating plan does; developing and administering a rating plan; promotion and upgrading; seniority and ability in promotions; other policy elements and promotions, handling promotions; disputes over promotions.

5. Transfer, downgrading and layoff—types of transfers; transfer policy; skill in handling transfers; downgrading versus layoff; use of rating in downgrading and layoffs; formulating a layoff policy; other aspects of layoff policy; employment stabilization.

6. Discipline and discharge—foundations of constructive discipline; formulating plant rules; types of disciplinary action; informing employees of disciplinary policy; "talking it over"; a situational approach to discipline; taking disciplinary action; discharge as a last resort; elements of the discharge policy.

7. Wage policies and wage administration—relation of wages to the

personnel program; the general level of wages; making wage surveys; other factors affecting wage levels; internal wage and salary relationships; job description analysis; elements of job evaluation; advantages of job evaluation; limitations and problems in job evaluation; advancing individuals within the rate ranges; responsibility for wage and salary administration.

8. Methods of wage payments: output standards—the personnel administrator's role; basic method of wage payments; employee attitudes on wage incentives; requirements of a good wage incentive system; group and plant-wide incentive; getting employee acceptance of new output standards; sharing the gain: the place of profit sharing; annual wage and guaranteed employment plans.

9. Hours of work and shifts—optimum hours of work; trends in working hours; payment for overtime work; responsibility for rescheduling hours; shift operation; characteristics of different shifts; meeting shift problems; rest and meal periods; paid vacations and holidays.

10. Services for employees—the scope of employee services; how should services be offered; services in a large company; limitations necessary for mutual protection; special services; questions to be asked in considering a program.

11. Employee health and safety—policies for health and safety; planning for health; organization for safety; organization for health; the safety director's qualifications; his place and function; accident analysis; safety committees; relation to other personnel activities.

12. Employee participation and production problems—employee interest in production problems; suggestion systems and their requirements; acting upon suggestions; joint suggestion committee; limitations of a suggestion system; meetings with supervisors on improving efficiency; joint labor-management committees; union-management cooperation on production problems, and conditions necessary for its success.[6]

A recent survey of the activities of some 50 personnel departments in hospitals and homes in New York is presented in Exhibit 1.

Exhibit 1[7]

Functions	Total Responsibility (Assigned to Personnel Dept.)	Shared responsibility (Not Assigned Exclusively to Personnel Dept.)	Not Responsible or N/A
(1) Employment Non Professional	53	1	4
Professional (Including R.N.'s)	19	33	7
(2) Wage and Salary Admin. Position Recommend.	35	16	8
Job Evaluation	44	8	7
Salary Recommendations	42	11	6
(3) Training	22	21	16
(4) Benefits Administration	44	9	6
(5) Personnel Policy Formulation and Administration	44	10	5
(6) Labor Relations: Grievance Procedure	41	11	7
Arbitration	22	9	28
Contract Administration	22	9	28
(7) Employee Discipline	23	29	7
(8) Employee Recreation and Activity	34	15	10
(9) Employee Counseling	33	20	6
(10) Organization Planning: Charts	18	25	16
Table of Organization	22	26	11
Preparation of Budgets	11	39	9

To support such a broad spectrum of responsibilities, personnel departments have grown in size. Exhibit 2 displays the personnel ratios of these hospitals and homes. Personnel ratio is the number of employees involved in the personnel function for each 100 employees of the institution. In those institutions reporting, with total employment of 1,000 to 1,999, the personnel department had .51 employees for each 100 employees.

Until quite recently, the personnel function in health care facilities was accepted as a necessary evil by the busy, parochial and task-oriented admin-

Exhibit 2[8]

PERSONNEL RATIOS

Number of Employees	Personnel Ratios, (per 100 employees)
1 - 999	.49
1,000 - 1,999	.51
2,000 - 2,999	.44
3,000 & over	.53
MEDIAN	.50

istrator. The growth of sophisticated and professionally sound personnel departments in such institutions has been the product of several forces:

1. Pressure from outside forces that have brought the fear of God into the health care milieu, i.e., union organizing efforts.

2. Pressure from the public and governmental agencies to effect cost reductions and controls over expenditures in the face of spiraling costs.

3. Internal pressures from within the organization to meet the multi-faceted employee relations problems brought to the fore by virtue of increased exposure to management literature, high turnover rates, employment of marginal workers and undemocratic, uneven treatment of employees.

4. Employment of "sleeper" personnel administrators innately motivated to do more than employment work.

The personnel department is no longer an employment department; the personnel manager is no longer an employment manager. In today's health care institution, the personnel department assists the director and his operating associates in planning for the growth of the organization, developing the organization to carry out the overall objectives of the institution and the controlled measuring of results. In this last area, the personnel department acts as deputy to the chief executive by performing the following functions:

1. Setting standards (the personnel staff is usually responsible for gathering information by which operations and performance can be measured and evaluated).

2. Measurement (particularly in the area of turnover, absenteeism and accidents).

3. Evaluation (attempts to quantify performance).[9]

It is important to note that the activities of the personnel department are directed toward making line control of the human element stronger and more effective—not toward usurping that control.[10] The personnel department *assists* the hospital administration, *advises* the hospital administration and *aids* the hospital administration. The personnel director is a resource individual. With his department and staff he provides surveys, analyses, information—all directed toward implementing the effective utilization of manpower.

One must recognize the difference between the line and staff function; it is most important to accept the fact that the personnel function is staff. The line carries the responsibility for action. The staff functions are essentially advisory and supplementary. The staff counsels, advises and assists the line. Its major responsibilities are the formulation of policy, consultation to the line and, above all, service to the line.

Placement of the Personnel Department
in the Institution's Organizational Structure

Personnel executives feel strongly about the place of their department in the institution's hierarchy. It is suggested that the department report directly to the director of the institution. A survey stated a twofold rationale for this position:

1. Placing the personnel executive at the top promotes better company (institution) decisions by encouraging all executives to give weight to personnel factors in their decision-making.

2. It enhances the personnel manager's professional status since this position reflects the importance the company (institution) attaches to his function. With sufficiently high status, the personnel executive can urge the establishment of new programs and carry out existing ones more successfully.[11]

In another study of 249 companies of all types and all sizes, 161 of the personnel departments reported directly to either the chairman of the board or president of the company.[12] More often than not the personnel department is perceived quite differently by members of the top administrative group of the institution as compared to a department head, operating supervisor or rank-and-file employee. The personnel department is viewed as a much more potent force at the operating level than at the top administrative level. Opinions of personnel decline markedly with the ascent of the management hierarchy. [13] Many top-level executives feel that the personnel manager is not sufficiently aggressive and innovative while others find him infringing upon their areas of responsibility. The latter look at the personnel department as a passive research function which should keep out of the way of the top administration. The former see the personnel executive and his department as the creative and innovative group which must institute new ideas, suggestions or recommendations advising top management and providing feedback as to programs and their effect upon the organization. [14]

Jobs in the Personnel Department

Titles for the top personnel executive in health care facilities vary considerably. The most prevalent one is that of personnel director. Some health care institutions designate their top personnel executive as personnel manager, personnel administrator, director of human resources, director of industrial relations, chief of personnel, associate director for personnel or assistant director for personnel. A few institutions use the title of vice-president for their key personnel executive.

Jobs that report directly to the top executive of the personnel department are the wage and salary administrator, the labor relations manager, the employee relations manager, the manager of training and the employment manager. Lesser positions include managers of personnel research, safety, employee services, employee counseling and employee benefits. In other subsections of the personnel department one finds such positions as job analyst, employment interviewer, personnel statistician, personnel assistant and personnel clerk. A more recent development places the management engineering and electronic data processing responsibilities within the control of the key personnel executive.

Personnel Administration as a Profession

It is not unusual within the context of the hospital and general health care facility environment to appreciate the drive toward identification of the personnel function as a profession. Many health occupational groups still cling tenaciously to outdated role conceptions. [15] In a setting with so many professions already recognized as such, the personnel administrator is hard-pressed to gain recognition for his role as a professional. It has been suggested that such efforts may best be appraised by considering what appear to be essential qualifications of a profession.[16]

1. Each profession has a *specialized terminology*—a professional "universe of discourse."

2. Each profession requires special knowledge and skill as a basis for the uniform performance of *standard practices and procedures*. These practices are voluntarily understood and accepted by members of the profession as ap-

propriate under given circumstances.

3. These practices are based on specialized training and on conscious research and study.

4. All professions assume the sharing of information among members of the profession—the opposite of the "patent medicine" or "trade secret" practice of some nonprofessional groups.

5. All professions maintain a continuous flow of *professional literature,* the principal purpose of which is to disseminate information on current experiments, discoveries and developments.

6. All professions require a high degree of *personal responsibility* on the part of managers, coupled with a similar freedom and independence of action.

7. All professions require for membership certain *standards of ethical practice.*

8. All professions require of their membership *primary allegiance to the profession,* to a code of ethics and to the public interest.

The growing demand for professional recognition, although an understandable sign of the times, may well be a two-edged sword. Professional recognition can be an incentive for quality performance. On the other hand such recognition, once a sign of competence and determination to excel, may soon be regarded as evidence of acquisitiveness and status-seeking. Often in the name of improving performance standards, professional or quasi-professional groups have introduced rigid credentialing requirements and have effectively lobbied for inflexible licensing laws. Each occupational group in its attempt to achieve professional status has effectively increased the educational requirements to gain entry into the inner sanctum. The model for professionalism in hospitals is the physician.[17] Each of the emerging professions wants to become its own "force" and is sensitive to interference by any other profession or by the administration. By isolating themselves in enclaves, they complicate the organization needed to operate the hospital efficiently.

The personnel director more than any other person must be extremely sensitive to the inherent anti-administration facets of the drive for professionalism. The acceptance of personnel administration as a profession goes far beyond certification, education and membership in associations. In the final analysis, it is the competence of the individual holding that responsibility which will lift the status of the profession.[18]

Conclusion

Personnel executives are key members of the top administrative group in an institution. Most decisions made in health service facilities involve people. The management of people is a personnel function. Each supervisor, each administrator and, yes, each physician in numerous ways is involved in managing manpower. The role of the personnel department is to effect agreement from administration as to the systems and processes that should serve as the context within which personnel decisions are made; to administer and monitor these systems and processes; to provide expert opinion on the development and administration of the systems and processes; and to participate as one of the top administrative groups involved in making personnel decisions. [19] The personnel department and its chief executive in a health service facility are involved in organizational planning and control, job analyses, job evaluation, wage and salary administration, recruitment, screening and selection, testing, employee performance evaluation, communications through employee handbooks and policy manuals, training and development, suggestion systems and the administration of fringe benefits. Each of these will be discussed in subsequent chapters.

Notes

1. George Ritzger and Harrison M. Trice, *An Occupation in Conflict: A Study of the Personnel Manager* (Ithaca, N.Y.: New York State School of Industrial and Labor Relations, Cornell University, 1969), p. 6.

2. Heckmann and Huneryager, *Management of the Personnel Function* (Columbus, O.: Charles E. Merrill Books, Inc., 1962), p. 3.

3. Henry Eilbert, "The Development of Personnel Management in the United States," in Heckmann and Huneryager, *op. cit.,* p. 20.

4. *Ibid.,* p. 16.

5. Malcolm T. MacEachern, "Functions of the Personnel Department: Hospitals are People," *Hospital Organization and Management* (Chicago: Physicians Record Company, 1957), p. 961.

6. Paul Pigors and C. A. Myers, *Personnel Administration* (New York: McGraw-Hill, 1947), pp. 20-21.

7. Reprinted from Grover Clark, Robert C. Grillo, and Norman Metzger, "Salaries, Ratios, Personal Data and Organizational Responsibility in Personnel Administration in Voluntary Hospitals," in *Profile: Hospital Personnel Administration–1967 (Journal of the Association of Hospital Personnel Administrators,* January, 1968).

8. Reprinted from *Journal of the Association of Hospital Personnel Administrators,* January, 1968.

9. "Personnel Administration: Changing Scope and Organization," *Studies in Personnel Policy,* No. 203 (New York: National Industrial Conference Board, 1966), p. 18.

10. "How to Establish and Maintain a Personnel Department," No. 4 (New York: American Management Association, 1953), p. 12.

11. Dalton E. McFarland, "Company Officers Assess the Personnel Function," No. 79 (New York: American Management Association, 1967), p. 27.

12. "Personnel Administration," *op. cit.,* p. 15.

13. Ritzger and Trice, *op.cit.,* p. 71.

14. *Ibid.,* pp. 64-75.

15. Eleanore C. Lambertsen, "Outdated View of Professional Function Is Bar to Better Care," *The Modern Hospital* (June, 1967), p. 142.

16. Dale Yoder, *Personnel Principles and Policies* (Englewood Cliffs, N.J.; Prentice-Hall, Inc., 1957), pp. 45-46.

17. Frederick Herzberg, *Work and the Nature of Man* (New York: The World Publishing Company, 1966), p. 184.

18. Harvey L. Smith, "Two Lines of Authority: The Hospital's Dilemma," *Modern Hospitals* (March, 1955), pp. 59-64.

19. Ritzger and Trice, *op. cit.,* p. 75.

ADDENDA

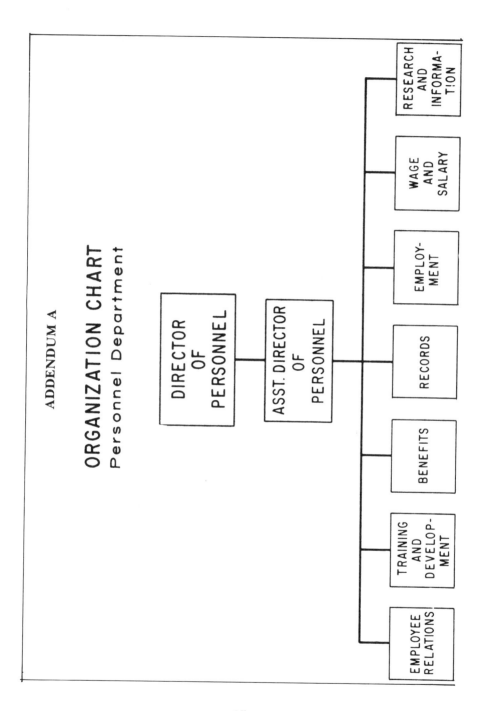

ADDENDUM A

ORGANIZATION CHART

Personnel Department

DIRECTOR OF PERSONNEL

ASST. DIRECTOR OF PERSONNEL

EMPLOYEE RELATIONS

TRAINING AND DEVELOP- MENT

BENEFITS

RECORDS

EMPLOY- MENT

WAGE AND SALARY

RESEARCH AND INFORMA- TION

ADDENDUM B

PERSONNEL DIRECTOR

Job Duties

Plans, coordinates, and administers policies relating to all phases of hospital personnel activities:

Plans and develops a personnel program and establishes methods for its installation and operation. Develops the techniques and procedures for and directs the activities of recruitment, induction, placement, orientation and training. He may also be responsible for the safety and security programs. Interprets hospital policies and regulations to new employees, arranges for their physical examinations, and conducts or advises on training programs. Establishes uniform employment policies and confers with department heads and supervisors to discuss improvement of working relationships and conditions. Assists in development of plans and policies related to personnel and advises supervisors and administrative officials regarding specific personnel problems. Initiates and recommends policies and procedures necessary to achieve objectives of the hospital and insure maximum utilization and stability of personnel. Initiates and directs surveys related to turnover, wages, benefits, morale, and other personnel considerations. Prepares training manuals and directs job analysis program, including preparation of job descriptions and specifications. Acts as liaison between employees and administrative staff. Investigates causes of disputes and grievances and recommends corrective action. Supervises workers engaged in carrying out personnel department functions.

Plans and sets up system of recordkeeping. Devises forms relative to the personnel functions. Organizes system for maintenance of central personnel files that will provide ready analysis of all personnel management functions.

Administers benefit services and other employer-employee programs, including recreation, pension and hospitalization plans, credit union, vacation and leave policies, and others. Initiates and implements employee suggestions and performance evaluation systems.

Informs employees of hospital activities and administrative policies by means of handbooks, house organs, bulletin boards, and other media. Performs research as a basis for recommending changes in procedures and policies. Interviews all terminating employees to determine causes of termination. Represents hospital at conferences relative to personnel activities. Prepares budgets.

Machines, Tools, Equipment, and Work Aids

Office supplies and equipment.

Education, Training, and Experience

Graduation from a recognized college or university with a degree in personnel management, industrial relations, or business administration.

Courses should include tests and measurements, statistics, applied psychology, personnel and business administration, economics, labor relations, and cost accounting.

Experience as Assistant Personnel Director is recommended. Receives inservice indoctrination in hospital policies and regulations.

Worker Traits

Aptitudes: Verbal ability is required to discuss personnel programs with administrative staff and employees of varying levels of verbal ability, to effectively promote the personnel program, and to explain hospital policy to individuals and groups. Capability also required to prepare manuals.

Numerical ability is required to evaluate personnel statistical data, to make various computations of departmental operations, and to prepare budgets.

Clerical ability is required to avoid and detect errors in verbal and tabular material prepared for submission to administrative personnel.

Interests: A preference for technical activities in order to develop and administer personnel policies.

A preference for activities that involve working with people in order to make the personnel policy effective and satisfactory to all hospital employees and to administrators.

Temperament: Ability to direct and plan the activities of the entire Personnel Department.

Ability to communicate with hospital staff and outsiders as well as workers within his department, in making and carrying out personnel policies and regulations.

Must be able to make decisions.

Physical Demands and Working Conditions: Work is sedentary, requiring lifting and handling personnel records and files, seldom exceeding 10 pounds.

Frequent talking and hearing when conferring on personnel matters, interviewing, or assigning work to subordinates.

Works inside. Usually has own office.

Job Relationships

Workers supervised: Employment Manager; Interviewer; Training Officer, Job Analyst; and clerical staff.

Supervised by: Administrator.

Promotion from: Assistant Personnel Director or Employment Manager.

Promotion to: No formal line of promotion. May be promoted to an Associate Administrator.

Professional Affiliations

American Society for Personnel
 Administration
52 East Bridge Street
Berea, Ohio 44017

American Personnel and Guidance
 Association
1605 New Hampshire Avenue, N.W.
Washington, D.C. 20009

Public Personnel Association
1313 East 60th Street
Chicago, Ill. 60637

American Society for Hospital
 Personnel Directors
840 North Lake Shore Drive
Chicago, Ill. 60611

State and local personnel associations and societies.

ADDENDUM C

TRAINING OFFICER

Job Duties

Assists in planning, organizing, and directing employee training programs designed to orient employees, improve job skills, and develop potential capabilities:

Confers with supervisors and department heads to determine need for training in order to increase job proficiency or improve morale. Plans new or special training classes and demonstrations, writes training material or adapts existing materials to immediate needs. Prepares and distributes pamphlets, memoranda, or manuals to be used by trainees. Schedules classes in cooperation with department heads, and arranges for lectures, demonstrations, or on-the-job training. Orients new employees to hospital policies, methods, and procedures.

Institutes supervisory training programs to develop more effective relationships between supervisors and subordinates. Instructs supervisors and department heads in training methods and use of training materials, and assists other members of the department with specific training or personnel problems.

Instructs employees relative to nature and hazards of equipment and materials handled, responsibilities of specific positions, and hospital safety rules. Conducts or arranges for sessions for introducing new procedures or equipment. Follows up program to evaluate effectiveness of training and to determine need for revision of methods or materials.

Selects and edits training materials such as educational films and books for training purposes. May prepare handbooks outlining personnel policies of institution, including information relative to salary and promotion; insurance, vacation, sick leave, and other benefits; standards of what is expected of employees and what they can expect from the hospital.

Designs training charts and other visual aids.

The duties of this job may be combined with those of Interviewer, Job Analyst, Employment Manager, or Personnel Director.

Machines, Tools, Equipment, and Work Aids

Audiovisual equipment, training manuals, and other aids.

Education, Training, and Experience

Graduation from accredited college or university with courses in educational methods, personnel administration, applied psychology, English and possibly journalism.

Teaching experience or experience in personnel work is essential.

Inservice training in hospital procedures and routines.

Worker Traits

Aptitudes: Verbal ability is needed to communicate (on a teacher-student basis) with workers of varying cultural and educational backgrounds and to prepare manuals and training materials.

Clerical perception is needed to organize and prepare manuals and training materials.

Interests: A preference for activities concerned with people and the communication of ideas to them.

A preference for activities concerned with creating effective training materials.

Temperament: Suitable for work that involves a variety of conditions to conduct a meaningful instructional program geared to the needs of the hospital.

Ability to communicate with people in actual job duties, beyond giving and receiving instructions, when orienting them to hospital and giving on-the-job training.

Influences people through ideas of training and accident prevention programs.

Physical Demands and Working Conditions: Work is light. Sitting when preparing materials and standing when conducting training sessions.

Talking and hearing when conducting training sessions.

Near-visual acuity for reading and writing training materials.

Works inside.

ADDENDUM C *(Cont'd)*

Job Relationships

Workers supervised: None.

Supervised by: Personnel Director.

Promotion from: No formal line of promotion. May be promoted from Interviewer.

Promotion to: No formal line of promotion. May be promoted to Personnel Director after additional training and experience.

Professional Affiliations

American Society for Personnel
  Administration
52 East Bridge Street
Berea, Ohio 44017

American Personnel and Guidance
  Association
1605 New Hampshire Avenue, N.W.
Washington, D.C. 20009

Public Personnel Association
1313 East 60th Street
Chicago, Ill. 60637

ADDENDUM D

INTERVIEWER

Job Duties

Interviews and screens job applicants to determine qualifications for employment with the hospital:

Conducts initial interviews of applicants for employment. Assists applicants in filling out application forms and requests additional information or clarification of data as necessary. Answers questions and supplies information regarding employment policies and requirements. Notes appearance, manner, and experience of applicants and other requirements of hospital employment policy. Refers qualified applicants to Employment Manager. Checks references on applications to verify work history. Receives requisitions for personnel from various departments, and refers qualified applicants from names in file, or contacts various sources to obtain workers.

Prepares reports supplying information on present employees or new employees, as requested, Maintains personnel records and makes changes necessary to keep records up to date. May administer and score tests not requiring special education and training.

The duties of this job may be combined with those of Employment Manager, Job Analyst, or Training Officer.

Machines, Tools, Equipment, and Work Aids

Office supplies and equipment; test forms.

Education, Training and Experience

Graduation from approved college or university with courses in personnel or business administration and psychology.

Should be.skilled in interviewing techniques.

Inservice training in hospital policies and personnel procedures and routines.

Worker Traits

Aptitudes: Verbal ability is required to communicate with applicants and department heads to successfully place workers in available jobs and to administer and evaluate tests.

Numerical ability is required to prepare and interpret statistical reports on job functions, in relation to recruitment, interviewing, and placement.

Clerical perception is required to organize pertinent details of verbal and written material.

Interests: A preference for business contacts, to place present and future employees in satisfactory and satisfying jobs.

A preference for activities concerned with communicating to explain the policies and regulations of the hospital to candidates for employment.

Temperament: Ability to communicate with applicants, to understand and provide help for their employment problems.

Ability to collect, organize, and interpret data from personal interviews, application forms, tests results, and letters of recommendation to assist in making proper placement.

Physical Demands and Working Conditions: Work is sedentary with some lifting and carrying of personnel files.

Reaches for and handles records and reports.

Frequent talking and hearing are required in communicating with applicants, and with other hospital workers.

Works inside.

Job Relationships

Workers Supervised: None.

Supervised by: Employment Manager.

Promotion from: No formal line of promotion.

Promotion to: Employment Manager.

Professional Affiliations

None.

ADDENDUM E

700	
Classification #	
531	Personnel
Department #	Department Name
1-S	
Grade	

POSITION DESCRIPTION

Personnel Administrator A
Classification Title

January 10, 1974
Date Prepared

Wage and Salary Manager
Position Title

Date Revised

Exempt
FLSA Status

Duties Performed:

Non-Bargaining Unit
BU Status

Conducts internal and external surveys of job tasks, salaries, policies and procedures in order to ensure and maintain equitable, competitive wages and working conditions for union and non-union employees. Determines relationships among jobs for purposes of transfers and promotions.

Performs job audits, interviewing employees to determine the nature of job functions; working conditions; tools and equipment used and job related educational/experience job requirements. Utilizes data collected to establish and maintain a classification structure of jobs, titles, salary grades and rates of pay.

Writes job descriptions outlining job content, lines of promotion and summary of salient job features. Estimates cost impact resulting from promotions, transfers, reclassifications and other positional and/or employee changes.

Evaluates the need for computerized reports by meeting with the request originator, Personnel Director and EDP Analyst. Determines the criteria necessary to produce reports with EDP programmers. Delivers reports explaining report content, format and coding.

Plans computerized personnel reports production and systems with Systems Analysts and Programmers. Ensures that Medical Center policies are followed in the development of the Personnel Information System, which provides positional and employee information in various formats. Reviews and evaluates requests for revision to Personnel Information System from user departments including changes in design, scheduling and report format.

C.4.E.5 Rev.
MSH 11-71 2M

24

ADDENDUM F

POSITION DESCRIPTION

700	
Classification #	
531	Personnel
Department #	Department Name
1-S	
Grade	

Personnel Administrator A
Classification Title

January 10, 1974
Date Prepared

Employee Relations Manager
Position Title

Date Revised

Exempt
FLSA Status

Non-Bargaining Unit
BU Status

Duties Performed

Gives advice and recommends alternate courses of action to department heads, managers and supervisors in the handling of employee relations problems.

Interprets union contracts and hospital policy for department heads, managers and supervisors.

Supports and fosters the principle of industrial justice for all medical center personnel.

Conducts third step grievance hearings.

Conducts formal training programs for supervisors in basic supervisory skills, human relations aspects of supervision.

Assists in preparation of arbitration cases. (Fact finding, briefs witnesses, reviews testimony).

Maintains informal channel of communication with medical center personnel.

Counsels non-bargaining unit personnel on job related problems.

Makes recommendations to Personnel Director on the need for policy changes or the initiation of new ones.

Conducts orientation sessions of new employees.

Assists in preparation of cases before the Human Rights Commission.

ADDENDUM G

ORGANIZATION OF THE PERSONNEL FUNCTION	Issued: 11/1/70
Page 1	Revised:

The following outline describes the functions, responsibilities and organization of the Personnel Department. It is designed to familiarize the reader with the resources available to him in dealing with personnel matters. However, one important fact should always be kept in mind: although the Personnel Department recommends policy and provides essential services, it is the departmental supervisor who is ultimately responsible for personnel administration in his unit.

3.1 Personnel Functions - The Personnel Department performs the following functions: Employement, Labor Relations, Employee Relations, Employee Counseling, Training and Development, Wage and Salary Administration, Personnel Records, Employee Benefits, Employee Housing, Personnel Communications, Research and Policy.

    3.11 Employment:

        3.111 Recruit, screen, test and place employment applicants.
        3.112 Cultivate recruitment resources.
        3.113 Conduct employment interviews.
        3.114 Place employment advertisements.
        3.115 Facilitate transfer of employees.
        3.116 Process newly hired employees.
        3.117 Assure compliance with hiring regulations.

    3.12 Labor and Employee Relations:

        3.121 Prepare for and conduct collective bargaining negotiations.
        3.122 Resolve grievances; represent Mount Sinai at grievance arbitrations and at hearings of government agencies.
        3.123 Advise on disciplinary matters.
        3.124 Assure compliance with personnel policy, collective bargaining agreements, and labor and civil rights laws.
        3.125 Coordinate employee activity and recreation programs.
        3.126 Recommend programs to improve employee motivation and performance.

II. JOB ANALYSIS AND
JOB DESCRIPTIONS

The need for scientific wage determination in any enterprise, including hospitals and homes, is well-established. Wage rates in the health care industry have risen to unprecedented heights through a spiraling succession of negotiations and pressures, both market and societal. Although wages may not be the key to motivation (and indeed one despairs at the absence of a concomitant rise in efficiency when wages are raised) employee dissatisfaction about wages is quite pronounced in hospitals and homes. This dissatisfaction has two separate causes:

1. Inequities among wage rates paid within classifications and in classifications employees consider similar to their own.

2. Individual or group pressure for higher earning power.

For many years hospitals and homes have been dealing with wages by fiat: an arbitrary order of importance is established and an arbitrary wage structure follows. This method is certainly eroded by group pressures from unions, professional associations and employees with skills which are in short supply. A sounder method of establishing wages is through job evaluation. The central purpose of job evaluation is threefold: to determine the relative worth of the various jobs in the institution; to establish a wage scale which incorporates fair differentials among jobs; and finally, where necessary, to correct pay inequities.

Job evaluation serves three major purposes:

1. Wage rates which will be defensible can be established on a quasi-scientific and logical basis. They are thus removed from the world of conjecture, arbitrariness and subjectiveness.

2. The bane of health care administration, *personalized rates,* will be abolished. Consequently, select pressure groups so prevalent in most hospitals and homes will be neutralized. No longer will the administrator be faced with the problem of misclassifying the secretary to a chief of service who protests that his secretary should receive as much as the secretary to the director of the institution.

3. Job evaluation is a key tool for the administration in attempting to meet competition by establishing a formal wage pattern that will conform

27

with health care wage rates in the area and, in general, with community wage rates.

To fully appreciate and understand the worth of job evaluation, one must consider the entire process from inception to fruition. The components of a job evaluation program include:

1. Job analysis.
2. Job descriptions.
3. Job specifications.
4. Job evaluation.
5. Wage structures.
6. Wage and salary administration.

Job Analysis

Job analysis is the scientific determination through intensive study and review of the actual nature of a specific job. It involves a study of each of the tasks which make up a job, including the skills, knowledge, abilities and responsibilities required of the worker. Its earliest origins can be traced to the time and motion studies first developed by Frederick W. Taylor in 1881 at the Midvale Steel Company. Taylor's use of analysis was directed toward determining a standard time for production. The purpose of motion study was pointed toward improving the methods of performing jobs. Industrial engineers look to eliminating unnecessary elements of the job and simplifying those that must be done. The industrial engineer conducting a time/motion study approaches it from the point of view of the job operation by observation and timing. He studies the sequence of operations, notes the machines and equipment involved and observes the movements of the worker in detail. His purpose is to improve the sequence, establish standards, simplify the work and conserve effort. Time and motion studies, however, do not provide the most complete answer to wage determination.

Job analysis, on the other hand, merely takes the job *as it is*, describing the duties, responsibilities, working conditions and relationship to other jobs, and does not involve itself with possible changes in the operation. The National Personnel Association in 1922 defined job analysis as "that process which results in establishing component elements of a job and ascertaining the human qualifications necessary for its successful performance." This definition sees job analysis as establishing job elements, which truly is the job of the industrial engineer. A more modern connotation envisions job analysis as reporting what currently exists in a job and *not* establishing job elements. There are basically three steps in the analysis of any job:

1. Identifying the job completely and accurately.

2. Describing the task of the job.

3. Indicating the requirements for its successful performance.

In the first step of job analysis, *identifying the job*, a specific job must be distinguished from every other job in the organization. It must be given a title and its geographic location must be clearly indicated. In describing the duties and responsibilities of the job, one is concerned with such factors as where the work comes from, what the worker does to it and what mental and physical processes are necessary for completion of the job. When the duties and responsibilities of the job are identified, the approximate time that each is performed must be indicated. In analyzing the skill and physical requirements, one must be concerned with mental skills—education, judgment, initiative—and manual skills—dexterity and motor skills. The physical requirements include such factors as standing, sitting, reaching and lifting. The working conditions and job hazards direct attention to the general environment in which the job is performed.

Definition of Terms

At the outset, it is necessary to define some of the terms common to the process of job evaluation.

Job: A job is made up of tasks and responsibilities which, when considered as a whole, are regarded as the regular assignment of the individual employee.

Occupation: An occupation is a group of closely related jobs which have many characteristics in common; however, each job of the occupation has its individual characteristics.

Position: Many employees may work at the same job. Each employee is said to be occupied in a position. For example, the job of porter in a hospital may be filled by 50 individuals who occupy 50 positions.

Job description: A job description is a written report including the duties and conditions to be found in a specific job.

Job specification: A job specification is a section of the job description which addresses itself to the personal requirements, skills and physical demands of the job.

Uses of the Job Analysis

Job facts are secured through the process of job analysis for many reasons. Some of these end products follow:

Job evaluation: Job analysis and job evaluation are not synonymous. Job evaluation is an end result of a job analysis. It establishes a foundation upon which a plan can be implemented to determine basic wage and salary differentials. These salary differentials are based upon the relative differences in job requirements.

Selection and placement: Job analysis results in job descriptions and specifications which provide an orderly and effective guide for matching applicants to positions in the interviewing procedure. Appropriate tests may be developed as a result of job analysis results. The job specification developed from the job analysis breaks down the job into its various components and, more importantly, details the qualifications necessary for jobholders.

Performance evaluation: Once again the job description developed from the job analysis may be used, this time to quantify specific elements to be measured on the job—standards against which an employee may be rated. These specific criteria for the successful jobholder may be used as a guide for merit rating.

Training: Job analysis can provide detailed information that serves as a basis for the training department's development of curriculum.

Labor relations: Job analysis provides a specific breakdown of duties that can be used to answer grievances regarding the nature of the employee's responsibilities. Job analysis, producing a job description, serves as a means of developing a mutual understanding between the administration, the union and employees regarding the specific duties of each job. It may eliminate or reduce grievances regarding pay differentials if the analysis is used to produce a scientific job evaluation.

Wage and salary survey: Job analysis provides a method of comparing rates of jobs in one institution with those in another.

Organizational analysis: Job analysis can clarify lines of responsibility and authority by a detailed breakdown of each job. It can indicate functional, organizational positioning of jobs.

The Job Analyst

A threshold decision must be made as to who will conduct the job analysis. There are three basic sources from which job analysts may be selected:

1. Employees within the institution.
2. Personnel supplied by consulting firms.
3. Personnel recruited from outside the institution.

Notwithstanding the source from which the job analyst is obtained, he (she) must have the ability to get along with others and be able to maintain an objective point of view. The analyst must write clearly and concisely, analyze and interpret diverse data and, in many instances, work on his own. It is essential that he obtain a high degree of cooperation from employees and supervisors in areas where he will be studying jobs. Upon this degree of cooperation rests the success of the entire program. It has been said that the only way to learn job analysis is by doing it. Although many college-level courses incorporate the subject of job analysis within the rubric of overall personnel administration, the person involved in the field must receive intensive training as to the organizational structure, its nuances and the personalities involved. It is obvious that choosing an employee presently in the employ of the institution has many advantages. He will know the organization, be familiar with its operating procedures, traditions and mores, and have a good understanding of the personalities involved. He is more likely to be accepted than the outsider who suffers from the suspicions of others as to his ultimate role.

Steps in the Design of the Program

Several steps must be taken to ensure the success of a job analysis program. First, the development of the plan; second, the presentation of the plan to top administration; third, the presentation of the plan to the supervisory group; and finally the presentation of the plan to the nonsupervisory group.

Development of the Plan

Careful planning is the hallmark of the successful job analysis program. The first decision to be made is the method of conducting the analysis. Each of the methods, their advantages and disadvantages, will be discussed later in this chapter. Marketing is probably the most important aspect to be considered in the planning stage. Obtaining employee and supervisory participation is essential. Methods of presenting the program to the administration, supervision and rank-and-file employees must be carefully developed. The selection of job analysts and their training is still another aspect to be considered in the planning stage.

Presenting the Plan to Top Administration

The acceptance by top administration of the need for and worth of a job analysis program is essential in assuring the success of that program. In order that the top administration may have facts upon which to make its decision with regard to authorizing a job analysis study, a complete presentation covering the various phases of the program and outlining in depth the steps to achieve the desired results must be made. Such a presentation to the director and his immediate staff should include such items as:

1. The nature of job analysis.
2. The main objectives of the program.
3. Why the organization will benefit from such a program.
4. Reference to the experience of other institutions preferably in the same field with such programs.
5. The cost of the programs.
6. Cost savings to be derived from such a program.
7. Who will conduct the program.
8. The methods to be used in assembling the information.

Presenting the Plan to the Supervisory Group

A combination of approaches can be used in presenting the proposed job analysis study to the supervisory group. Some of the more prevalent and successful methods are:

1. Staff meetings.
2. Individual meetings with supervisors.
3. Memoranda from the top administration to the supervisory group.

The combination of any or all of these methods is not unusual. The program will not suffer from overcommunication. Full and broad publicity will aid in its acceptance and guarantee its results. To reduce problems that result from suspicions and lack of understanding on the part of the supervisory team, maximum participation of supervisors must be obtained. They must understand the complete method of job analysis and the hoped-for results. This requires an educational program wherein the basic nature and philosophy of a job analysis program are communicated. Strong emphasis should be placed on the benefits to the supervisors from such a program. In general, supervisors will be reluctant to spend the time required to implement a job analysis program unless they first accept and acknowledge that there will be positives for them which develop from such an endeavor. In addition, it is wise to assign to each supervisor a specific responsibility as part of the program. The supervisor himself may be responsible for explaining the procedures to the employees. As described later in this chapter, the supervisor may well fill out the job analysis questionnaire or aid the employee in completing the form. In either case, it is essential that he be made to feel a part of the program and not an outsider.

Presenting the Plan to the Nonsupervisory Group

The fourth cornerstone in ensuring the success of the plan is the full understanding and cooperation of the employees in the institution. They must understand *why* such a program is necessary and the benefits that will accrue to them from the program. Letters to the employees from the administrator, group meetings with employees, individual interviews with employees and departmental meetings led by supervisors all play a role in obtaining maximum cooperation of the nonsupervisory group. It is a well-established principle that employees want to know what is going on and want to participate in effecting change. Any assumption that employees are not interested in an explanation of a new program is an invalid one. The need to feel a part of things is a pervasive one. A program such as this should not be legislated; it should be "sold" to the employees. Communication, once again, is the key to this marketing procedure. In addition, it is best to introduce the job analyst to the employees in advance to facilitate and ease the analyst's job.

Training the Analyst

Once the analysts who will conduct the program are selected, various methods or combinations of methods are used to train them. Among these are:

1. A study program involving literature that is widely available.

2. Lectures and conferences during which the analysts are presented the details of *what* they are to do and *how* they are to do it, and a careful review of the forms to be used.

3. Role playing during which the analysts conduct practice interviews, followed by a critique and a refinement of the techniques.

It is important that the analyst understand the advantages to the institution of such a program. He must be instructed in the method of completing the information on a questionnaire, in conducting interviews with supervisors and with employees and in methods of obtaining information through observation.

Not the least of the training essentials is in the area of writing drafts of the data assembled. The style of writing such drafts must be as uniform as possible. It is on the basis of such information that job descriptions are developed. Therefore, a terse, direct style must be employed, and all words that do not impart necessary information to an understanding of the job duties should be omitted.

How to Collect the Data

There are basically three methods of obtaining information about jobs:

1. The analyst may make use of a questionnaire sent to the job incumbent, who fills it in, has it checked by his supervisor and returns it when completed.[1]

2. The analyst may interview the worker or the supervisor or both to

obtain the necessary information.

3. The analyst may collect the data from personal observation.

A discussion of each of these methods follows.

Questionnaire Method

This is the most rapid and economical of the methods. The worker or the supervisor or both complete a questionnaire which covers all phases of the job, its environment and overall responsibilities. The questionnaire is then returned to the job analyst who carefully reviews it for content and completion and edits it in preparation for the writing of a job description. The preparation of the questionnaire is critical to the success of this method. It must be carefully prepared to solicit all the pertinent facts about the job and, therefore, must indeed be universal in application since most job analysis programs include varying and disparate jobs. In the development of a questionnaire, the use of check boxes can reduce to a minimum the writing required of the employee. A closer review of the contents of a job information form and the typical subdivisions of such a questionnaire follow (see Exhibit 1):

1. The employee's name, the department, his present position, job classification and date of preparation.

2. Description of duties (job content) with approximate percentage of time applied to each duty. This section calls upon the employee to describe the duties and responsibilities of his position. He is asked to include enough detail and use language that will clearly convey the content and requirements of the position to a person not familiar with the work. He is asked to describe regular ongoing activities and then periodic or occasional duties. He must make estimates of the frequency with which each duty is performed, e.g., daily, weekly, monthly, and approximate percentage of working time normally consumed on each of the duties.

3. The educational requirements of the job. Include the minimum education normally required to perform the work satisfactorily. It does not follow that the incumbent's present educational background coincides with the requirements of the position.

4. Experience requirements. Here the employee is asked to indicate the nature and extent of experience required for an individual with the specified educational background to perform the work satisfactorily. This includes previous experience and necessary break-in time with the present employer.

5. The employee is asked to describe the degree of supervision ex-

Exhibit 1

LAURRIET PRINTING CO., INC.

THE MOUNT SINAI HOSPITAL
JOB INFORMATION FORM

A.   **B.**

REVIEW REQUESTED BY _____ DATE _____   DEPARTMENT _____ SECTION _____

PURPOSE OF REVIEW: CURRENT JOB CLASSIFICATION _____

☐ TO CLASSIFY NEW POSITION

☐ TO ASCERTAIN WHETHER JOB CHANGES REQUIRE   POSITION OR FUNCTIONAL TITLE _____
  RECLASSIFICATION OF POSITION.

☐ TO ASCERTAIN WHETHER ESTABLISHED   EMPLOYEE'S NAME _____ EMPLOYEE # ____
  CLASSIFICATION IS APPROPRIATE

☐ DEPARTMENTAL JOB AUDIT.   POSITION #(S) _____

☐ OTHER: _____   PREPARED BY _____ DATE _____

                                                     APPROVED BY _____ DATE _____

C. JOB CONTENT – DESCRIBE THE DUTIES AND RESPONSIBILITIES OF THE POSITION. INCLUDE ENOUGH DETAIL AND USE LANGUAGE THAT WILL CLEARLY CONVEY THE CONTENT AND REQUIREMENTS OF THE POSITION TO A PERSON NOT FAMILIAR WITH THE WORK. DESCRIBE REGULAR, ONGOING ACTIVITIES FIRST, THEN PERIODIC OR OCCASIONAL DUTIES. INDICATE THE FREQUENCY WITH WHICH EACH DUTY IS PERFORMED (E.G., DAILY, WEEKLY, MONTHLY), AND THE APPROXIMATE PERCENTAGE OF WORKING TIME NORMALLY CONSUMED.

	FREQUENCY	APPROXIMATE % OF TIME

PAGE 1

Exhibit 1 *(Cont'd)*

C. __JOB CONTENT__ (CONTINUED) —

	FREQUENCY	APPROXIMATE % OF TIME

DESCRIBE THE MOST CRITICAL OR COMPLEX ASPECTS OF THE WORK, DIFFICULT SITUATIONS THAT MUST BE DEALT WITH, UNUSUAL DEMANDS THAT THE INCUMBENT MUST SATISFY, AND SPECIALIZED KNOWLEDGES, SKILLS, TECHNIQUES, AND EQUIPMENT THAT MUST BE UTILIZED.

Exhibit 1 *(Cont'd)*

H. CONTACTS WITH OTHERS – DESCRIBE THE RESPONSIBILITY TO SERVICE, DEAL WITH, OR INFLUENCE OTHER PERSONS.

WITH WHOM?	INDIVIDUALS DEALT WITH	PURPOSES OF CONTACTS	FREQUENCY
☐ EMPLOYEES IN OWN DEPARTMENT			
☐ EMPLOYEES IN OTHER DEPARTMENTS			
☐ DEPARTMENT HEADS			
☐ ADMINISTRATIVE OFFICIALS			
☐ MEDICAL STAFF			
☐ PATIENTS			
☐ VISITORS			
☐ OUTSIDE OFFICIALS			
☐ OTHERS			

I. RESPONSIBILITY FOR CONFIDENTIALITY – IF POSITION ENTAILS WORKING WITH CONFIDENTIAL DATA (E.G., MEDICAL REPORTS, FINANCIAL STATEMENTS, PERSONNEL RECORDS), DESCRIBE NATURE OF DATA, DEGREE OF CONFIDENTIALITY, AND EFFECTS OF DISCLOSURE. DESCRIBE PRECAUTIONS THAT MUST BE TAKEN TO KEEP THE INFORMATION SECURE.

J. PHYSICAL DEMAND – DESCRIBE THE PHYSICAL EXERTION REQUIRED TO PERFORM THE WORK. HOW OFTEN, AND WITH WHAT CONSTANCY DOES THE WORK REQUIRE STANDING, WALKING, LIFTING, REACHING, STOOPING, PUSHING, ETC.?

K. MENTAL, VISUAL AND MANUAL COORDINATION – DESCRIBE THOSE ASPECTS OF THE WORK THAT REQUIRE ATTENTION TO DETAIL, CONCENTRATING ON CRITICAL PROCEDURES, OVERCOMING DISTRACTION, COORDINATING SIMULTANEOUS OPERATIONS, AND EXERCISING MANUAL DEXTERITY.

L. RESPONSIBILITY FOR EQUIPMENT OR PROCESS – INDICATE THE PROBABLE DOLLAR VALUE OF CARELESS DAMAGE TO EQUIPMENT OR LOSS OF TIME BECAUSE OF INCORRECT PERFORMANCE OF A WORK PROCESS. DESCRIBE THE SITUATIONS IN WHICH SUCH LOSSES ARE POSSIBLE.

$ _____

M. RESPONSIBILITY FOR MATERIALS – INDICATE THE PROBABLE DOLLAR VALUE OF A TYPICAL LOSS DUE TO CARELESS WASTE OR SPOILAGE OF MATERIALS OR SUPPLIES. DESCRIBE THE SITUATIONS IN WHICH SUCH LOSSES ARE POSSIBLE.

$ _____

N. RESPONSIBILITY FOR SAFETY AND WELFARE OF OTHERS – DESCRIBE THE EXTENT TO WHICH CARE MUST BE EXERCISED TO PREVENT INJURY, DISCOMFORT, OR IMPAIRMENT OF HEALTH OF OTHERS. INDICATE POSSIBLE ACCIDENTS RESULTING FROM MISUSE OF EQUIPMENT, MISMANAGEMENT OF MEDICAL CARE, ETC.

Exhibit 1 *(Cont'd)*

O. **RESPONSIBITY FOR WORK OF OTHERS (NON-SUPERVISORY POSITIONS ONLY)** – CHECK THE STATEMENT THAT MOST CLOSELY DESCRIBES THE EMPLOYEE'S RESPONSIBILITY FOR INSTRUCTING, GUIDING, OR ASSISTING OTHERS IN THEIR WORK:

- [ ] RESPONSIBLE SOLELY FOR OWN WORK
- [ ] RESPONSIBLE FOR LEADING UP TO TEN EMPLOYEES IN WORK GROUP
- [ ] RESPONSIBLE FOR MAINTAINING WORK FLOW OF MORE THAN 25 EMPLOYEES
- [ ] RESPONSIBLE FOR INSTRUCTING, GUIDING, OR ASSISTING ONE OR TWO EMPLOYEES
- [ ] RESPONSIBLE FOR MAINTAINING WORK FLOW OF UP TO 25 EMPLOYEES

P. **WORKING CONDITIONS** – DESCRIBE SURROUNDINGS IN WHICH WORK IS PERFORMED

_____

_____

INDICATE DISAGREEABLE CONDITIONS PRESENT IN WORK AREA, E.G., HEAT, COLD, DAMPNESS, FUMES, NOISE, DUST, DIRT, ETC., AND WHETHER EXPOSURE IS CONSTANT, FREQUENT, OR OCCASIONAL.

_____

_____

Q. **UNAVOIDABLE HAZARDS** – DESCRIBE ACCIDENT AND HEALTH HAZARDS INCIDENT TO WORK EVEN THOUGH ALL POSSIBLE SAFEGUARDS ARE OBSERVED.

_____

_____

R. **SUPERVISION OF OTHERS (SUPERVISORY JOBS ONLY)**

CHARACTER OF SUPERVISION: LISTED BELOW ARE A VARIETY OF ADMINISTRATIVE AND SUPERVISORY FUNCTIONS. INDICATE IN THE APPROPIATE COLUMN THE DEGREE OF RESPONSIBILITY AND AUTHORITY WITH WHICH THE EMPLOYEE ACTS IN EACH FUNCTION. USE THE FOLLOWING DEFINITIONS AS A GUIDE:

- NA – NOT APPLICABLE TO THIS POSITION.
- 1 – HAS AUTHORITY TO ACT ONLY AFTER APPROVAL BY SUPERVISOR.
- 2 – NO AUTHORITY TO ACT BUT HAS RESPONSIBILITY TO RECOMMEND ACTION AND TO IMPLEMENT ACTION AFTER APPROVAL IS RECEIVED.
- 3 – HAS FULL AUTHORITY TO ACT WITHOUT PRIOR APPROVAL BUT MUST ADVISE SUPERVISOR AFTER ACTION IS TAKEN.
- 4 – HAS FULL AUTHORITY TO ACT WITHOUT CONSULTING SUPERVISOR BEFORE OR AFTER ACTION IS TAKEN.

FUNCTION	NA	1	2	3	4
PLAN WORK SCHEDULES					
ASSIGN WORK TO EMPLOYEES					
REVIEW COMPLETED WORK					
INSTRUCT EMPLOYEES ON THE JOB					
DEVELOP TRAINING PROGRAMS					
DETERMINE STANDARDS OF PERFORMANCE					
APPRAISE EMPLOYEE PERFORMANCE					
REPRIMAND EMPLOYEES FOR FAILURE TO MEET PERFORMANCE STANDARDS					
DISCIPLINE EMPLOYEES FOR INFRACTION OF REGULATIONS					
INVESTIGATE AND RESOLVE GRIEVANCE					
SELECT APPLICANTS FOR EMPLOYMENT					
DISCHARGE EMPLOYEES FOR UNSATISFACTORY PERFORMANCE					
RECOMMEND SALARY ACTION					
RECOMMEND PROMOTION OR TRANSFER					
GRANT TIME OFF					
AUTHORIZE OVERTIME					
APPROVE SUPPLY REQUISITIONS AND PETTY CASH EXPENSES					
PURCHASE CAPITAL EQUIPMENT					
PREPARE AND MAINTAIN BUDGET					
DEVELOP AND IMPLEMENT IMPROVED METHODS AND PROCEDURES					
DIRECT PATIENT CARE OR ACTION					
OTHER: (DESCRIBE)					

ercised over his position and guidance available to him in performing his task.

6. The impact of errors. The employee is asked to describe the results of errors possible from improper performance of the work.

7. A description of the responsibility for contacts with others such as employees in his department and in other departments, department heads, medical staff, patients, visitors and outside officials.

8. If his position entails working with confidential data, the employee is asked to describe the nature of the data, the degree of confidentiality and the effects of disclosure. He is asked to describe precautions that must be taken to keep the information secure.

9. Physical demands. Here the employee is asked to describe the physical exertion required to perform the work. How often and with what frequency does the work require standing, walking, lifting, reaching, stooping or pushing.

10. Mental, visual and manual coordination. A description of the aspects of the work that require attention to detail, concentrating on critical procedures, overcoming distraction, coordinating simultaneous operations and exercising manual dexterity.

11. Several sections deal with responsibility for equipment or process, for materials and for safety and welfare of others.

12. Working conditions. The employee is asked to describe the surroundings in which the work is performed and to indicate disagreeable conditions present in the work area, such as heat, cold, dampness, fumes, noise, dust and dirt, and whether exposure is constant, frequent or occasional.

13. Unavoidable hazards. A description of accident and health hazards incident to work even though all possible safeguards are observed.

14. In the case of supervisory jobs, the character of the supervision exerted. The supervisor is asked to describe the degree of responsibility and authority which he applies to other employees.

15. Scope of supervision. Here the supervisor is asked to indicate the number and types of employees directly and indirectly supervised.

Advantages of the Questionnaire Method

The questionnaire method is the most rapid for obtaining information. Time is often a prime consideration, and by using questionnaires distributed to the employees whose jobs are to be described, more jobs can be analyzed than by the interviewing method in the allotted time. It ensures maximum participation of employees since by its very nature a questionnaire can be sent to a large number of employees without the involvement of too much of their own time as well as the time of the administration. It has the distinct advantage of channeling employee thinking regarding their jobs because of the well-planned format of the questionnaire. In the final analysis it is one of the least costly methods of obtaining job information. An adjunct advantage reported by one observer is that problems dealing with cross-divisional responsibilities can be identified and corrected.[2]

It is well to note that all advantages of the questionnaire method stem from the design of the questionnaire. The critical element in the success of this method is the specificity of the questionnaire, and often institutions have developed separate questionnaires for clerical, technical, professional and service jobs.

Disadvantages of the Questionnaire Method

It is almost impossible to design a questionnaire that will bring forth complete information on all jobs. Because of the varying backgrounds of employees who are asked to fill in questionnaires, terminology is often inconsistent, and therefore interpretation of the questionnaire is difficult at times. Hourly and clerical employees often are ill-equipped to write paragraphs or answer questions that will give the analyst the necessary information to describe the job.[3] This method requires extensive editing of information. Experience with questionnaires indicates that often they must be supplemented by interviews to clarify information and complete responses. Low-level personnel do not take the time to provide extensive, clear and complete information about their job duties. The absence of personal contact minimizes the chances for employee understanding of the program. It has been noted that some employees resent the questionnaire approach and suspect that their job rate might depend on what they write and not on what they do.[4]

Interviewing Method

In obtaining job analysis data, the analyst may interview either the supervisor or the employee involved in doing the job, or both. The analyst usually has a plan or guide to follow in his questioning and can get more complete and accurate information regarding a job in an interview than would usually be obtainable through any other method. The procedure is quite simple. First, the analyst observes the worker on the job while he is performing a complete cycle. He will than ask any questions that arise about any specific part of the operation. The analyst takes notes, often copious in nature, indicating the areas which he has failed to grasp or questions which he may have about a specific aspect of the job. He will then study the information that he has noted to check for continuity of data. He will talk directly with the worker and/or the worker's supervisor. Often it is wise to recheck the worker's comments and the analyst's notes with the supervisor. It is essential that the worker be informed during the interview and observation stage that he must perform his job in the usual manner.

Good interviewing in job analysis is quite similar to effective interviewing in other aspects of personnel work. Of course, the purpose is quite different: securing a patterned or preplanned set of job facts. An important secondary purpose is that of winning the understanding, cooperation and interest of the employees and supervisors interviewed. Patton, Littlefield and Self suggest a guide for job analysts during the interviewing procedure:[5]

1. Introduce yourself; review briefly the purposes of the analysis; give any individualized explanation needed; answer questions.

2. Follow your interview guide or work-sheet form in asking questions, but recognize that the various items of information will not always come out in any set order.

3. Phrase questions clearly and follow through with each until a full understanding is reached.

4. Use a high degree of tact and show interest in anything the employee has to say. Be a careful listener.

5. Avoid making promises or giving expressions of opinion regarding the probable value of the job at this stage and avoid making suggestions as to possible improvements in working methods.

6. Write up the job just as you find it, disregarding both the ability of the employee on the job and any previous notions which you may have had regarding the job. If you think erroneous information has been given, make notes and check later but do not directly question the truth of the interviewee.

7. Assure the employee that you will let him check and verify the description before it is written up in final form.

8. Thank the employee for his cooperation.

Advantages of the Interviewing Method
More than any other method, interviewing permits the analyst to secure complete and accurate information. It obviates the employees having to complete questionnaires at home if their jobs do not provide facilities for work of this nature and also avoids the necessity for employees to describe their work in writing, which is often very difficult for employees with little

background in such a skill. The personal touch is a decided asset in explaining the program and winning employee understanding. Editing and standardizing language is minimized since the analyst is carefully trained in writing his observations from the interview. By firsthand interviewing and observation, the analyst is able to accurately reduce the information to the more essential aspects of the job.

Disadvantages of the Interviewing Method

This method requires a great deal of time when a large number of jobs must be analyzed. Therefore, it is relatively expensive because the salaries of both the analyst conducting the interview and the employee (who may well be less productive during that stage) are involved. Because of the time and expense, this method is usually applied to a limited number of employees and does not provide for the broad participation which is the hallmark of the questionnaire method.

Observation Method

This method is quite similar to the interview method except that the analyst only observes the operation and does not question the employee. Rarely used on its own, it is often combined with the interview method or the questionnaire method. During the observation method the analyst makes notes, avoids disturbing the worker and carefully observes the "what, how and why" of the skill involved and the physical demands of the job. He then reviews his notes, attempting to assure continuity of operation. His primary concern is to discern the factual information from judgment or impression. It has been said that the chief characteristic of the scientific method is the requirement that the observer be trained to distinguish what he observes from what he would like to infer. This indeed is the crux of the observation method. Its disadvantage lies in the fact that it would be quite difficult to apply this method for operations that require mental skills to a large degree, as well as to operations which are long-run and, therefore, must be observed over long periods of time.

Observation and Interview: Combined Method

After reviewing the advantages and disadvantages of the observation method and the interview method, it is not difficult to deduce that by combining these two methods most of the disadvantages are minimized and the advantages maximized. The analyst would first obtain as much information as possible by observing the job without disturbing the worker. After reducing his observations to notes, he would interview the supervisor and the worker to supplement facts. This would ensure the assembling of information which could not be obtained by observation and provide the mechanism to verify and augment those facts obtained by observation.

During the observation method the analyst makes notes, avoids disturbing the worker and carefully observes the job as it is being done. He then reviews the notes with the worker and the supervisor to fill in where necessary and to modify impressions which may not be based upon the actual elements of the job.

The Mechanics of Job Analysis

The following is a typical plan for implementing a job analysis.

1. Visit department head:

a. Explain the purpose and objectives of the plan.

b. Discuss the desired method for obtaining the information, e.g., questionnaire, observation, interview.

c. Make maximum effort to obtain the understanding of the department head and, therefore, his cooperation.

d. Secure a list of all the jobs in the department by title and the number of employees in each title. (This information can be obtained in advance from the personnel department and verified with the department head.)

2. With the approval of the department head, visit the supervisor and/or assistant supervisor:

a. Explain the purposes and objectives of the plan.

b. Obtain an overview of the work of the section.

c. Discuss the specific job in question with emphasis on the nature of the work and the details of the job.

d. Obtain recommendations of the most desirable employees to observe during the course of the study on the basis of efficiency and willingness to cooperate with the analyst.

3. Observe employees at work:

a. Carefully note each operation performed.

b. Make certain all observable operations have been noted.

c. Separate judgment or impression from factual information.

d. Check for specific items to be included in the job analysis schedule.

e. Report factual data of working conditions, equipment and materials used.

f. Question the worker about those operations which are not observable and obtain from the worker an estimate of the percentage of time such operations are performed.

g. Review the notes concerning the job elements with the worker, ask for suggestions and obtain from him an estimate of the percentage of time each operation is performed.

4. Review observations and notes with assistant supervisor and/or supervisor:

a. Determine if the job has been thoroughly covered.

b. Obtain estimates of percentage of time for each operation. (Check these estimates against the estimates noted from comments of the employee.)

c. Obtain information as to the relationship of this job to other jobs in the section.

5. Write the first draft of the analysis in prescribed format.

6. Have department head review and approve the original draft:

a. Allow all supervisors concerned the opportunity to review and edit the original draft.

b. Revise draft on the basis of comments, changes and criticisms suggested by the reviewers and obtain written approval of contents before final typing.

c. Arrange for typing of the completed analysis—one copy to be retained in the analysis file, one copy to be forwarded to the wage and salary administrator, one copy to be forwarded to the personnel director and one copy to be forwarded to the department head.

Job Descriptions

No single instrument is as important to effective wage and salary administration as the job description, yet there is evidence that it receives far less attention than it requires to assure either that it is properly prepared in the first place or that its uses are properly understood or directed.[6]

The process of obtaining job facts through job analysis moves to the next critical step: the writing of a statement of the duties, responsibilities and job conditions. Having completed the task of assembling all the requirements of a specific job, the job analyst has at hand, through a questionnaire, notes from an interview or direct observation, all the pertinent items which make up the regular assignment of an employee on an individual job. Having conducted a job analysis, he has in front of him the following information: the objective of the job, including its basic mission and what it accomplishes; to whom the incumbent reports; how many people he supervises; what levels and types of positions report directly to the incumbent; which areas and operations are included in the position; to what extent the incumbent is responsible for actions and decisions, completely or partially; whether his actions are subject to approval from his supervisor; the extent to which he is responsible for results; the type of planning involved in the job; other units of the institution which are directly affected by this planning; the relationships of the incumbent in the job to other departments within the institution and others outside the institution; the extent and nature of his responsibilities for policy interpretation; the procedures and methods to be followed; and specialized technical information required to handle the job.

The analyst is now prepared to write a job description. *A job description is a listing of the duties and responsibilities of a particular job, written in narrative form.* Its content and style may vary considerably, based upon the end to which it will be used. There is a guideline which may be followed when the description is to be used for the standard purpose of job evaluation, training and/or planning. An effective job description has four basic subdivisions: *"heading," "job summary," "duties performed"* and *"personal requirements."* Patton, Littlefield and Self offer the following principles as a guide to writing effective job descriptions:[7]

1. Arrange duties in logical order. If a definite work cycle exists, duties may be described in chronological order. When the work cycles are irregular, more important duties may be listed first, followed by less important ones.

2. State separate duties clearly and concisely without going into such detail that the description resembles a motion analysis.

3. Begin each sentence in the "duties performed" section with an active, functional verb in the present tense, such as "tests," "performs," "adjusts," etc. For brevity, the subject of each sentence is omitted. It is understood that the job title is the subject.

4. Use quantitative words where possible. Rather than "pushes loaded truck," write "pushes hand truck loaded with 100 to 500 pounds of steel plates."

5. Use specific words where possible. Instead of writing that a patternmaker "makes" patterns, write that he "saws stock to length on circular saw and roughly to width on ripsaw; shapes with woodworking machines and hand tools." Avoid vague words and ambiguous generalizations such as "handles," "assists" and "prepares," unless further information is given which makes the meaning specific. If the words fail to evoke a mental image of the work, rephrase using a more specific verb.

6. State duties as duties; postpone statements of qualifications until the "personal requirements" or "job specification" section.

7. Avoid proprietary names that might make the description obsolete when equipment changes occur. Write "operates automatic electric desk calculator" instead of "operates Friden calculator."

8. Determine or estimate the percentage of total time spent on each activity and indicate whether duties are regular or occasional. The description should not imply that the jobholder spends most of his time at a demanding task when, in actuality, it may be performed only 5 percent of the time. Be sure to define such words as "periodic," "occasional" and "regular."

9. Limit the use of the word "may" with regard to performance of certain duties. Rating committee members will want to know whether the duty is performed or not performed; they are often confused if the description states that the operator "may perform" the duty. Nevertheless, occasions arise when the use of "may" is justified toward the end of the duty section when a "saving clause" broadening the description of duties must be inserted.

Heading

The job in question must be differentiated from all others in the organization. Therefore, the selection of the appropriate title is essential. In addition, concomitant identifying information should be established such as the department in which the job is performed and a job code number. Two helpful sources in job identification are *The Dictionary of Occupational Titles* and *Job Descriptions and Organizational Analysis for Hospitals and Related Health Services*, both published by the United States Department of Labor, Washington, D.C.

The importance of selecting an appropriate job title should not be underestimated. Social behaviorists have pointed out repeatedly the important roles that status and recognition play in the motivation of employees. Not only should the selected title *distinguish* a job from every other job in the organization, it should also be fully *acceptable* to the incumbents. Very often a job may have a master or generic title which encompasses several functional titles. In addition to the master title, any alternate titles by which the job may be known should be listed in the "heading" section. The title, as far as possible, should be similar to one used in the past for that job in that institution. Optimally, it should be one that is commonly used throughout the health care industry. It should be set up in its natural form, not in inverted form: e.g., nursing technician, not technician—nursing. It should be brief and should indicate wherever possible the skill and supervisory levels involved. In addition to the department in which the job is assigned, the date the information is secured should be clearly indicated at the top of the form. This keys the reader into the timeliness of the information. Where possible, the job description heading should include the name of the supervisor responsible for the specific job and the current salary or range for the job. All of this may be contained in the code number, which may be made up as follows: a section for indicating the department, the number(s) for the generic type of job, the number(s) for the skill level and the number(s) for the position.

Job Summary

This section of the job description gives the reader an overall concept of the purpose, nature and extent of the task performed. It is also meant to show how the job differs generally from others in the organization. This is best accomplished by a brief statement which avoids generalities and precedes a detailed presentation of the duties. It aims to give immediate understanding to the reader of the nature of the job without a profusion of details. Otis and Leukart present five points in the writing of an effective "job summary" section:[8]

1. The statement should be as brief as possible and still encompass its purpose.

2. Words should be selected carefully to carry the maximum amount of specific meaning.

3. The statement should differentiate the job from all other jobs accurately enough to be used in classifying workers on the job.

4. The purpose of the job must be clearly stated.

5. The job summary must conform to the what-how-why job analysis formula.

The "job summary" section is not one which encompasses details, duties and responsibilities. It is generalized in nature and has as its avowed purpose the establishment of the uniqueness of the job. It must communicate the *central purpose of the job.*

Duties Performed

This section is a complete description of duties of the job and is often referred to as the *body* of the job description. Each duty must be written in logical work order. This may be done either by describing the duties chronologically or by combining those which are of a similar nature. The decision as to how to present the tasks should be dependent on which method creates the clearest presentation. When writing the "duties performed" section, it is important that the requirements not be based upon the incumbent since he may be overqualified or underqualified for the position. It is essential to state the *minimum* requirements for the *average* incumbent. A succinct, direct style should be used. Each sentence should begin with a functional verb: for example, "transports patients to and from operating or treatment rooms, sets up equipment, instruments and medications for surgeons." It is best to use the present tense to minimize the number of words to be used. The pitfall one finds too often in job descriptions is that they are unnecessarily protracted. On the other hand, it is essential that each important duty be described. The job analysis material should be reviewed carefully before writing the "job summary" section. Grady offers three important questions which should be answered in the affirmative upon review of the job analysis information:[9]

1. Have you indicated clearly the knowledge and skills required on the job?

2. Have you shown the responsibilities and authority inherent in the job?

3. Have you included a statement of working conditions?
He also makes the following suggestions in writing the "duties performed" section:[10]

1. Start each paragraph with an active verb.

2. Use telegraphic style (complete sentences are not essential, but making sense is).

3. Avoid the use of general words such as "maintains," "checks," "handles," "prepares," "takes care of" *unless* the level of work is further specified.

4. Make plentiful use of "such as" and "by doing" (one or two examples frequently are clearer than several sentences of description).

Personal Requirements
The "personal requirements" section or "job specification" section is concerned primarily with reflecting the skill involved and the physical demands of the job. It is used as the basis and justification of the values which will be assigned to each factor for the purpose of evaluating the job's worth. (Job evaluation programs and the selection of job factors will be described in detail in the next chapter.) It is used as well to facilitate selection and placement.

Since the most widely used job evaluation plan is the point-factor method, the specification under this plan would encompass from six to twelve specific factors. The most common factors found in a job specification are those for education, experience, initiative, ingenuity, physical demands, working conditions and unavoidable hazards. The job is then broken down into its requirements paralleling the job factors to be used in evaluating the job. The analyst must determine and describe the extent of each factor in the job. Once again each factor is described in terms of the *minimum* requirement for the *average* incumbent. For example, under the factor "education," a typical specification would include "ability to read or write and speak English, follow directions and make simple arithmetic calculations equivalent to four years of high school education." The specification for experience would include the years of experience necessary to perform the requirements of the position in a satisfactory fashion, e.g., "over seven years of progressive experience as a cook in a hotel, restaurant or hospital." Under the specification for working conditions, the description in a normal situation might read, "Works in a well-lighted kitchen; subject to burns and scalds from hot equipment and foods and injury from falls on slippery floors." Unavoidable hazards are included under the working conditions factor. In some instances specifications may be written separately for unavoidable hazards. All the specifications must be specific and quantitative. Patton, Littlefield and Self suggest several key principles in writing the specification section:[11]

1. Break down the job requirements parallel to the job factors to be used in evaluating the jobs. For each factor selected for use in the job evaluation plan, determine the extent of that requirement in the job being described.

2. Be as specific and quantitative as possible.

3. State the *minimum* requirement for the *average* jobholder. Avoid confusing a jobholder's personal qualifications with the minimum requirements of the job.

4. Distinguish between the job's minimum requirement and the hiring qualifications. A low-level job may require no more than the ability to read, write and do simple arithmetic. Yet the hospital may require all entering employees to possess a high school diploma to ensure their advancement.

5. Check to ensure that every duty corresponds to the requirements.

An effective job specification will go further than a mere mention of personal requirements. It will seek to provide measurements of each of those requirements. Many job specifications contain minimum scores which must be attained on both intelligence and mechanical aptitude tests.[12] The job specification contains substantiating data for each factor to be considered. These substantiating data are measured against the degree descriptions for each factor contained in the wage and salary manual (see Exhibit 2).

Updating of Job Description

It is imperative that once the job description for each job is carefully constructed that a system be developed for keeping it up to date. It is

Exhibit 2

MOUNT SINAI HOSPITAL
NEW YORK, NEW YORK

Personnel Department

JOB EVALUATION SPECIFICATIONS

Code No. ......211..............

Department(s) ....

....

Labor Grade ......9..H................

Job Title ......NURSING AUXILIARY.......................... Class...... A .... Total Points ..180..............

	FACTORS	SUBSTANTIATING DATA	Degree	Points
SKILL	EDUCATION	Ability to read and write and speak English follow written and verbal instructions and use simple arithmetic and equipment.	3	25
	EXPERIENCE	Previous experience in related auxiliary nursing work preferred. On-the-job training yields full productivity in 6 months to 1 year.	2	40
	INITIATIVE AND INGENUITY	Requires ability to work from detailed procedures in performing work. Must use tact and judgment in dealings with patients, nurses and staff. Receives close supervision.	2	25
EFFORT	PHYSICAL DEMAND	Lifts, pushes and carries equipment, wheels portable apparatus; turns, bends, reaches and pulls in handling patients and setting up equipment.	3	15
	MENTAL OR VISUAL DEMAND	Must be mentally and visually alert during surgery and administration of treatments. Requires manual dexterity in setting up equipment and administering treatments.	3	15
RESPONSIBILITY	FOR EQUIPMENT OR PROCESS	Probable damage to equipment or instruments is negligible because of close supervision.	1	5
	FOR MATERIALS	Probable loss of materials and instruments is seldom over $10.00 because of immediate supervision.	1	5
	SAFETY OF OTHERS	Compliance with standard procedures and safety precautions essential in order to prevent accidents or cause further discomfort to patients.	3	15
	WORK OF OTHERS	Responsible for own work only.	1	5
CONDITIONS	WORKING CONDITIONS	Works in operating room and other patient-care surroundings.	3	15
	UNAVOIDABLE HAZARDS	Subject to burns and cuts from instruments, equipment and chemicals,and respiratory ailments from fumes.	3	15

REMARKS:

P-103

necessary to change the job description whenever significant changes are introduced into the job requirements. If such changes occur within the responsibilities of existing jobs, a new description must be written. It should be standard operating procedure for the line supervisor to inform the wage and salary manager of any significant changes to the job description and request an audit of the job. As a safeguard, many institutions schedule a periodic audit of all jobs in the organization. Each month the wage and salary section of the personnel department is responsible for auditing a specific number of jobs to update the job descriptions. Whenever a new job is created, there is a need to conduct a job analysis to produce a job description. This should be done at the outset. In fact, it is advisable to write the job description before an individual is hired for the new position. Brandt makes mention of specific changes which require the careful attention of the wage and salary section and alert them to the need for a revision of the present job description:[13]

1. A change in physical facilities or surroundings which might affect the comfort, fatigue or hazard factors of a job, creating or eliminating the need for protective garments or equipment and/or altering the way in which functions are performed.

2. A technological change might make the job easier or more difficult to perform. It might create or eliminate a need for special knowledge. It might also affect the time needed to perform a particular function so that the employee would be required to operate several machines or processes instead of one or the function might now be combined with other functions in order to fill out the job tour.

3. A change in supervisors might result in a realignment of several jobs into completely new combinations of functions which could entail an increase or decrease of difficulty and/or responsibility of any given job. Some of this restructuring might be a reflection of current interest or of a drive for more efficient use of manpower.

Conclusion

The job description has become indispensable to the process of classifying work into management components, for it is one of the important means by which the energy of the organization is unified in constructive channels.[14] Evans points out that "A clear line of demarcation can be drawn between a typical job description program for blue collar workers and that which is customarily found at managerial levels. Many survey respondents stated that they used their managerial position descriptions entirely for purposes unconnected with compensation rates. Rather . . . the principal goal of their program is to improve organization using the job description as a diagnostic tool to uncover defects."[15]

The job description plays an important role in administration as well as in manual positions within the organization. It is more than mere support for the salary program and may be used effectively in meeting performance standards. It has been stated that "when a manager and his subordinate are having an earnest discussion of some plan or decision affecting the subordinate's work, the conversation rests on the assumption that the two men are in fair agreement about the nature of the subordinate's job . . . If a single answer can be drawn from the detailed research study (presented in the report), into superior-subordinate communication on the managerial level in business, it is this: If one is speaking of the subordinate's specific job—his duties, the requirements he must fulfill in order to do his job well, his intelligent anticipation of future changes in his work, and the obstacles which prevent him from doing as good a job as possible—the answer is that he and his boss do not agree or differ more than they agree in almost every area."[16]

In order to ensure maximum agreement between superiors and subordinates, the administration must provide well-written job descriptions. These descriptions must then be widely publicized and complete agreement as to their content obtained from the supervisor and the incumbents in each job. The descriptions will be used to establish a foundation upon which to build a formal job evaluation plan and to provide an effective and objective guide for intelligent selection and placement as well as detailed information for inaugurating training programs. With proper quantification, the job descriptions will be used as a standard by which employees may be rated.

Notes

1. Charles W. Brennan. *Wage Administration* (Homewood, Ill.: Richard D. Irwin, Inc., 1963), p. 94.
2. Robert P. Vorhis, *"Collecting Data Through Questionnaires,"* in Milton L. Rock, *Handbook of Wage and Salary Administration* (New York: McGraw-Hill Book Company, 1972), p. 1-39.
3. *Ibid.*, p. 1-37.
4. *Idem.*
5. John A. Patton, C. L. Littlefield, and Stanley Allen Self, *Job Evaluation: Text and Cases* (Homewood, Ill.: Richard D. Irwin, Inc., 1964), p. 81.
6. Alfred R. Brandt, "Describing Hourly Jobs," in Milton L. Rock, *Handbook of Wage and Salary Administration* (New York: McGraw-Hill Book Company, 1972), p. 1-11.
7. Patton, Littlefield, and Self, *op. cit.*, pp. 93-4.
8. J. Lester Otis and Richard Leukart, *Job Evaluation* (Englewood Cliffs, N.J.: Prentice-Hall, Inc., 1948), p. 266.

9. Jack Grady, "How to Write a Job Description," *Job Evaluation and Wage Incentives* (New York: Conover-Nast Publications, 1949), pp. 66-7.

10. *Ibid.*, p. 66.

11. Patton, Littlefield, and Self, *op. cit.*, pp. 94-5.

12. Dale Yoder, *Personnel Principles and Processes* (Englewood Cliffs, N.J.: Prentice-Hall, Inc., 1956), p. 98.

13. Brandt, *op. cit.*, pp. 1-22

14. Gordon H. Evans, *Managerial Job Descriptions in Manufacturing* (New York: American Management Association, 1964), p. 13.

15. *Ibid.*, p. 19.

16. Norman R. S. Maier, L. Richard Hoffman, John J. Hooven, and William H. Read, *"Superior-Subordinate Communications and Management,"* No. 52 (American Management Association, 1961), p. 9.

ADDENDA

ADDENDUM A

JOB ANALYST

occupational analyst

Job Duties

Collects, analyzes, and develops occupational data relative to jobs, including job requirements and workers' qualifications, to serve as a basis for selection and placement of workers, wage evaluation, counseling, and other personnel practices:

In cooperation with department heads and Personnel Director, determines need for job analysis program, and procedures to be followed. Interviews workers and observes tasks being performed in order to identify job, describe duties, and indicate requirements for workers. Includes such pertinent information as use of equipment and tools; working conditions; and requirements for physical skills and knowledge, degree of dexterity, special sensory acuteness, and personal characteristics. Writes descriptions of each job emphasizing points of information needed for personnel practices involving recruitment; placement, promotion, and transfer; job and employee evaluation; training, full utilization of workers; safety and health research; improved personnel policies; and counseling. Reviews completed analysis with department head and Personnel Director for verification.

Writes hiring specifications to assist in making valid selection of prospective employees. Reviews job duties to reveal duplication of effort and establish promotion sequence of jobs. Devises employee performance evaluation criteria and job evaluation systems, and recommends changes in job classifications. May use tests to determine occupational knowledge and skill of worker. Determines interrelationships among jobs for purposes of transfer, promotion, and job redesign.

Assists in developing job analysis schedules and other personnel forms. Performs research to determine improved personnel procedures. The duties of this job may be combined with those of Interviewer, Training Officer, or Employment Manager.

Machines, Tools, Equipment, and Work Aids

Office equipment and supplies; testing and analysis forms.

LIBRARY ST. MARY'S COLLEGE

Education, Training, and Experience

Graduation from an accredited college or university, Courses in statistics, tests and measurements, and personnel administration are desirable. Experience in job analysis or similar phases of personnel work are essential.

Inservice training in hospital routines and procedures is provided.

Worker Traits

Aptitudes: Verbal ability is necessary to communicate with workers when making job studies, then to express clearly the details, so that the findings will correlate with the purposes of the job study.

Numerical ability is necessary to prepare wage and rating scales, statistical charts, and evaluation systems.

Clerical ability is necessary in preparing formats of personnel records and entering information on them.

Interests: A preference for technical activities, to support knowledge of equipment, terminology, and processes used by hospital workers.

A preference for activities of an abstract nature, for research to develop new personnel procedures, and to alleviate hospital personnel problems.

Temperament: Aptitude to collect, organize, and evaluate job data gathered from studies of hospital jobs.

Capable of making recommendations for improved use of personnel on the basis of evaluations made of job data.

Capability to meet and interview various types of workers and to observe duties being performed in all areas of the hospital.

Physical Demands and Working Conditions: Sits, stands, and walks intermittently throughout the working day.

Handles and fingers office supplies and equipment.

Talks and listens to employees when studying jobs.

Works inside.

Job Relationships

Workers supervised: None.

Supervised by: Personnel Director.

Promotion from: No formal line of promotion. May be promoted Interviewer.

Promotion to: No formal line of promotion. May be promoted to Personnel Director after additional training and experience.

Professional Affiliations

American Society for Personnel
  Administration
52 East Bridge Street
Berea, Ohio 44017

American Personnel and Guidance
  Association
1605 New Hampshire Avenue, N.W.
Washington, D.C. 20009

Public Personnel Association
1313 East 60th Street
Chicago, Ill. 60637

Source: Job Descriptions and Organizational Analysis for Hospitals and Related Health Services, (Revised Edition), U.S. Department of Labor--Manpower Division, 1971, pp. 172-3.

ADDENDUM B
JOB EVALUATION SPECIFICATIONS

Job Title...... LABORATORY TECHNICIAN .... Class.......... B ....

JOB DESCRIPTION:

GENERAL STATEMENT OF DUTIES:

Under general supervision, prepares and examines specimens following detailed, established laboratory procedures and records findings. Performs related duties.

WORK PERFORMED:

Performs one or more routine laboratory tests and procedures, such as, blood counts, urinalysis studies, preparation of histo-pathological specimens, culture and identification of microorganisms, chemical analyses, phlebotomizing donors, typing and handling blood units, assisting with animal surgery, preparing allergy test solutions, examining parasitology specimens, and, preparing EEG tracings.

Prepares, maintains, and records findings on records, charts and other special forms. Responsible for maintenance of order and cleanliness in laboratory area and equipment.

May perform other related duties as required.

Promoted From: USUALLY AN ENTRY JOB   Supervised By: LABORATORY
                     LABORATORY TECHNICIAN C,D   SUPERVISOR A, B

Promoted To: LABORATORY TECHNICIAN A   Supervision Over: LABORATORY
                                           TECHNICIAN (HELPER) D

May Be Identified As:

SENIOR TECHNICIAN	PART-TIME TECHNICIAN
TECHNICAL ASSISTANT	RESEARCH TECHNICIAN
NIGHT EMERGENCY LABORATORY	SPECIAL TECHNICIAN
TECHNICIAN	TECHNICIAN

60

ADDENDUM C

SALARY RATING SPECIFICATIONS

Position Title___NURSING AUXILIARY_____Class_____B_____

POSITION DESCRIPTION:

GENERAL STATEMENT OF DUTIES:

Under supervision, administers routine patient services, including personal hygienic and therapeutic procedures, and performs miscellaneous cleaning tasks. Performs related duties.

WORK PERFORMED:

Assists patients disrobe, put on Hospital clothing, and get in and out of bed. Transports patients by escorting, or pushing in wheel chair or on stretcher, to designated Hospital area. Answers call lights, handles bedpans, places side rails on beds, fills bedside ice and other containers and in general makes patient comfortable.

Bathes patients, prepares type of bath required, gives alcohol rubs, combs and washes hair, feeds and helps with general hygienic matters. Gives enemas and non-medicated care including steam inhalation as instructed, and application of ointments, and heat, using heat lamps.

Collects and disposes of body wastes. Measures, collects, records and describes specimens. Assists nurse in patient treatment by applying binders, hot or cold compresses and dressings, ice collars and hot waterbags. Takes, records, and charts temperatures, treatment, food, and fluid intake and output. May prepare nourishments, simple foods and serve patients.

Performs miscellaneous cleaning tasks, such as washing dishware, sterilizing instruments and equipment, making beds and dusting, cleaning and arranging furniture, storing linen on shelves, replenishing household supplies, emptying waste baskets, and collecting soiled wares and linen. Cares for patients' valuables and flowers. Assists in post-mortem care and runs errands.

May perform other related duties as required.

Promotion From: USUAL ENTRY   Supervised By: NURSE B, C, D, E
                JOB, NURSING
                AUXILIARY C

Promotion To: NURSING AUXILIARY A   Supervision Over: NONE

May be Identified As:

ATTENDENT   AIDE
ORDERLY   O. R. MESSENGER

III. JOB EVALUATION AND WAGE AND SALARY ADMINISTRATION

Fair wage and salary policies are essential to good industrial relations. If an organization were to formulate a statement of its industrial relations policies, it would probably conclude that compensation policy should be geared to achieve these two goals:

1. The general level of compensation should be consistent with the existing level for comparable jobs in the community or competitive hiring area.

2. Compensation for each job should be determined in relation to compensation for other jobs in the organization, with due regard for differences in knowledge and skill, responsibilities, and other factors significant to the general nature or type of jobs involved.[1]

The central objective of job evaluation is to determine the relative worth of each job in the institution. Once the relationship between jobs has been established, fair pay differentials must be designed, and finally any existing pay inequities must be corrected. There are three definitive and direct results which stem from a job evaluation program:

1. The institution can establish defensible wage rates arrived at on a quasi-scientific basis. Therefore, members of the union and administration have a factual, rather than an arbitrary basis for collective bargaining.

2. The personalized rate established by fiat (too common a practice in hospitals and homes) can be abolished. These rates often reflect pressures from the power brokers inside and outside the hospital.

3. Job evaluation can assist administrators in maintaining a position in the labor market which is competitive within their industry and their community.

Basic Steps in the Job Evaluation Ladder

The job evaluation program has eight basic steps:

1. Agree on the objectives to be attained and the jobs to be covered.

2. Select a job evaluation committee and the type of evaluation to be used.

3. Conduct a job analysis.

4. Convert the job analysis into a usable form.
5. Perform the evaluation.
6. Make a wage survey in the industry and the community.
7. Assign rates to each job.
8. Maintain the job evaluation program.

In establishing the objectives of the job evaluation program, certain policy decisions must be made. The cardinal purpose of the plan is to afford a basis for comparing different jobs. Wages, although a prime subject of these comparisons, should be considered a by-product. A more important objective is to establish the present relationship between jobs in the organization. Job requirements should be the basic determinants of the relative pay. The following policy decision should be made at the outset: no employee's rate of pay will be reduced as a result of the initiation of the job evaluation plan; on the other hand, underpaid jobs and employees will be given upward adjustments to conform with the findings of the evaluation. Another important policy which must be established—one which finds hospitals and homes in the role of the reluctant dragon—is that the general level of rates should be at least equal to or above the level prevailing in the locality and the industry.

Which Jobs Are to Be Evaluated?

In establishing objectives to be attained, it is important to identify which jobs are to be evaluated. A decision must be made on the groups of employees to be surveyed and the organizational level to which the study will be carried and whether or not the same evaluation plan should be used for all groups. Job evaluation is as applicable to high-level, high-paid jobs as to low-level, low-paid jobs. In recent years, institutions have used job evaluation for formalizing salary administration for the employed physician.[2] Limiting maintenance jobs, excluding supervisory, technical, professional and administrative jobs would be not only inadvisable but indefensible. It is not necessary to select the same type of job evaluation program for each of these groups. One may consider the more sophisticated Benge system (described later in this chapter) for professional jobs while using a point system for service and maintenance jobs. Job evaluation is applicable for all levels of responsibility in the institution.

Both the supervisors and the workers must be sold on the need for and value of job evaluation programs. Both groups should be fully exposed to all the advantages and implications of the program. A written communication describing the type of plan, the approach and the goals should be distributed to all employees. Supervisors must be made aware of the program's basic nature and philosophy. Their participation must be carefully planned and intelligently solicited. It is best to announce the institution of a job evaluation program in a letter to *all* employees explaining the objectives and methods to be used. Training sessions with supervisors should be held at an early stage.

The Job Evaluation Committee

The selection of the job evaluation committee and the evaluation method to be used are the most crucial and difficult elements of the entire program. In order to ensure the program's success, a representative committee is essential. In the average-sized hospital, the following people would make an excellent committee: the personnel director, director of nursing, building service manager, executive engineer and an administrative representative of the laboratories. It is important that the committee be as knowledgeable in the highest number of job areas as possible within the institution, although each of the members of the committee may well be a specialist. A parochial attitude and preconceived notions about the worth of other jobs in the institution are counterproductive. It is, therefore, essential that the committee members be impartial and analytical as well as objective. They must be liberal in their view of all jobs; otherwise, an attitude which is subjective and highly defensive can hinder the committee and result in long, personal arguments which tend to be diametrically opposed to the program's objectives.

Objectives of the Job Evaluation Plan

A job evaluation plan is the cornerstone of the compensation program of the institution. Before choosing the type of plan for a specific institution, it is important to adopt the basic objectives of the plan. Some of these objectives follow:

1. Pay employees at rates equal to or better than rates for positions requiring comparable skill, effort and responsibility in the industry and in the community.

2. Establish and maintain fair wage differentials between jobs in all departments in terms of the value of each job to the institution.

3. Pay all employees in accordance with all applicable federal and state legislation or regulations as to wages, hours and other conditions of work.

4. Follow the principle of equal pay for equal work assignments in the institution.

5. Recognize and reward employees based upon their individual ability, outstanding performance and length of service within the rate range established for the job occupied.

6. Develop a plan which is objective, simple and acceptable to the personnel affected.

7. Develop a plan which is flexible and adaptable to the unique needs of the institution.

Once the objectives of the job evaluation plan are established, a decision must be made as to the type of plan which will be used. The decision on the jobs to be covered affects the choice of the evaluation plan. For instance, it is well to repeat, it may be advisable that nursing positions be evaluated in a plan separate from that for service and maintenance positions. It is not uncommon to find two or three separate evaluation programs in operation in one institution.

Types of Job Evaluation Plans

The critical question of which type of evaluation program should be used and the design of such a program to fit the needs of the organization is the next order of business. There are four types of job evaluation plans: *the ranking method, the classification method, the point method* and *the factor comparison method*. The ranking and classification methods are nonquantitative in nature, while the point and factor comparison methods are quantitative. As indicated in Exhibit 1, the ranking method measures one job against another and in measuring the job it considers each as a whole.

Exhibit 1

CLASSIFICATION OF JOB EVALUATION SYSTEMS

	CONSIDERS EACH JOB AS A WHOLE	CONSIDERS EACH JOB ONE ELEMENT AT A TIME
MEASURES JOB AGAINST JOB	RANKING METHOD	FACTOR COMPARISON METHOD
MEASURES EACH JOB AGAINST A PRE-DETERMINED RATING SCALE	CLASSIFICATION METHOD	POINT METHOD

The classification method measures each job against a predetermined rating scale, and in so doing considers each job as a whole. The point method measures each job against a predetermined rating scale, but considers each job one element or factor at a time. The factor comparison method measures one job against another job, but considers each job one element or factor at a time. A detailed discussion of each of these methods follows.

The Ranking Method

This method considers each job as a whole and measures each job against every other. It attempts to establish an order of relative worth. Even with this very simple method, job descriptions are necessary. The jobs are not subdivided into factors; therefore, it is necessary to select committee members who have sufficient familiarity with a wide range of jobs. Several techniques can be employed to improve the accuracy of the ratings. Brief job descriptions may be posted on cards. Ranking is then completed by the method of paired comparisons. Each pair of jobs is compared and a decision is made as to which of the pair is more important. The number of comparisons to be made is $N(N-1)/2$, where N equals the number of jobs to be ranked. If an organization is using the ranking method and has determined that there are 100 jobs to be evaluated, the formula would be $100(100-1)/2$; thus, 4,950 comparisons would be necessary in ranking all jobs in the institution. It is helpful to begin with a small group of key jobs with which the committee is familiar and which have a going rate in alignment with the community and the industry. These key jobs would then be ranked and used as the point of comparison for all other jobs.

Another refinement of the straight ranking method is the factor-guided ranking technique. The evaluators rank job against job in terms of predetermined, defined factors, rather than by comparing whole job against whole job. Each factor, such as knowledge and physical effort, is ranked separately. When the evaluation is completed, there is a separate ranking for each factor. These rankings can be used to check the overall rankings of the *whole* job. This method helps sharpen the evaluators' judgment by focusing their attention on one factor at a time rather than on whole job comparisons. The evaluators, therefore, are less prone to subjective overall ratings.

More often than not, ranking is done on a whole job basis and by paired comparisons. Preconceived notions regarding prevailing pay levels, one's own work experience, personal observations and general notions as to training time required will almost inevitably creep in. It is not unusual for the evaluator to be biased by the title of the job. All of these disadvantages are reduced by using the factor-guided ranking technique. This slight extra effort tends to bring about considerably more accurate and consistent results. However, the ranking system can be an inaccurate method—difficult indeed because the organization may not have raters sufficiently familiar with a wide range of jobs. These disadvantages can be minimized by the selection of a competent evaluation committee, the availability of accurate job descriptions and the use of the factor-guided ranking technique. The advantages of this method are that it is simple to administer and explain to the raters, it requires little time to do the actual rating of the job and it is quite flexible. It can be effective in a small nursing home or small hospital where a limited number of jobs are being rated.

The Classification Method

The classification method is also known as the predetermined grading method. The evaluation is accomplished by preparing a set of job grades (with definitions for each grade) and classifying individual jobs in relation to how well they match the grade definitions. There are three steps to this method:

1. Job grades are established.
2. Each grade is carefully defined.
3. Individual jobs are classified in relation to the grade descriptions. The number of grades or classes established depends in part upon the institution's history, i.e., the number of job classes which have traditionally been used in the payment of workers. A minimum of six or seven grades can be established with a maximum of 17 to 20, although an optimum system appears to have 10 to 12 grades. The determination of the number of grades to be used in the grade description method depends upon such factors as:

1. The type of jobs to be included: e.g., clerical, administrative, professional, service and maintenance.
2. The range of salaries and wages paid: e.g., if there is a narrow range of wages paid for the jobs, less grades are necessary.
3. The range of skills involved in the job.
4. The institution's policy on promotion within a grade.

The key to the classification method is the grade description. Each grade description should contain the following general areas:

1. Type of work and complexity of duties.
2. Education necessary for performing the job.
3. Experience necessary for performing the job.
4. Supervision given and received.
5. Responsibilities.
6. Effort demanded.

A list of bench-mark jobs must accompany each grade description. These jobs serve as illustrations of the types of jobs which fit into this specific grade. At the core of the job classification method is the basic principle that within any given range of jobs there are differences in the levels of duties, responsibilities and skills required for performance.[2] Once these differences are established, a ladder can be established wherein each rung represents a different grade. Jobs are then assigned to the rung of the ladder which best fits their description.

A well-organized classification evaluation plan is made possible by the careful selection and definition of grade descriptions. When the number of grades has been determined, the evaluation committee is faced with the difficult but important responsibility of describing each grade. It is necessary to determine the general characteristics represented in the group of jobs to be classified. The grade definition does not follow an arithmetic scale; in fact, it is general and broad-based. It is designed primarily to reflect and cover the same basic elements present in all the jobs to be classified.

This type of plan is used by the United States Civil Service Commission. Each grade is covered under a general schedule; the lowest grade, GS1, includes the simplest, routine jobs which generally work under close supervision, while higher grades, such as GS17 and GS18, are jobs requiring broad latitude in judgment and high-level responsibility. The basic disadvantage of the predetermined grading method is the difficulty in developing grade descriptions which are generic yet will lend themselves to the classification of jobs in the organization. They tend to be too general. In addition, some jobs have tasks at many levels; therefore, part of the job, for example, would fall into Grade 2 while another might fall into Grade 4. On the other hand, it is a simple method of evaluation once bench-mark jobs are established and grade descriptions are carefully developed. It is easily understood, and since it is not a quantitative system containing complex and numerous factors, both raters and employees experience minimum difficulties in grading positions.

The Point Method

The point rating method is a quantitative system which measures a job by analyzed judgment against a predetermined rating scale. It does not measure the job as a whole but breaks the job down into various factors. This is the most widely used and accepted of all the evaluation systems. Each job is measured by comparing specific factors of the job with a predetermined rating scale. Essentially, it consists of a group of factors common to all jobs being rated, with a range of degrees for each factor. The different degrees are rated in points and the sum of the points assigned to a given job indicates its relative standing among the jobs being rated. There are four basic steps in a point rating job evaluation plan:

1. Each job must be studied to determine the factors which are generic in application for all jobs.

2. A determination must be made as to the number of degrees or levels needed to measure the presence of each factor in all jobs.

3. Each factor must be defined, as must each degree or level of that factor.

4. A weight must be assigned to each factor in proportion to its relative importance in the institution, as well as to each degree within that factor.

The most famous of the point rating plans was developed by the National Electrical Manufacturing Association and later adopted by the National Metal Trades Association. This plan uses anywhere from 5 to 12 factors (see Exhibit 2). There has been a trend in recent years to reduce the number of factors. Most institutions use separate plans for clerical jobs, executive jobs and service and maintenance jobs.

A typical point rating job evaluation plan would have factors for education, experience, complexity of duties, physical demands and working conditions. In selecting factors that may be universally applied to the jobs to be evaluated, the following criteria should be considered: the factor must be ratable, important, singular and universal in application, and it must point up a major characteristic which is common to all jobs. Each factor is divided into several degrees ranging from small to large. The number of degrees might differ for each factor. Only the number needed to measure the distinct levels of each factor should be provided. Therefore, under education, five degrees may be necessary, the lowest degree being *ability to read and write* and the highest degree *a university education;* the experience factor may need six degrees, the lowest described as *from up to and including three months of time usually required for a person to acquire the necessary ability to do the job* and the highest *requiring four years or more of experience.*

In constructing this type of plan, the selection of factors is the critical departure point. Deciding on which factors will be used is dependent on which jobs are to be evaluated. Once the jobs to be included under the job evaluation program are established, the major characteristics which are common to all those jobs must be determined. After outlining the characteristics which are common to all the jobs, their order of importance must be established. Since it is possible that many characteristics may be established which are present in most of the jobs to be evaluated, the number must be reduced to the minimum necessary to determine accurately the relative

Exhibit 2

POINTS ASSIGNED TO FACTORS AND KEY TO GRADES

FACTORS	DEGREES AND POINTS							
	1st	2nd	3rd	4th	5th	6th	7th	8th
1. Education	20	40	60	80	100	120		
2. Experience	25	50	75	100	125	150	175	200
3. Complexity of Duties	20	40	60	80	100			
4. Monetary Responsibility	5	10	20	40	60			
5. Contacts	5	10	20	40	60			
6. Working Conditions	5	10	15	20	25			
Add for Supervisory Jobs Only								
7. Type of Supervision	5	10	20	40	60			
8. Extent of Supervision	5	10	20	40	60			

POINT RANGE	GRADE
Up to 120	A
125-160	B
165-200	C
205-240	D
245-280	E
285-320	F
325-360	G
365-400	H
405-440	J
445-480	K
485-520	L
525-560	M

Source: National Electrical Manufacturing Association Job Evaluation Plan.

worth of each job. In doing this, the factors selected must be singular; they should not overlap other factors and should be the measure of one aspect of the job. They must be easily defined and understandable. Of course, the major characteristic of a factor to be selected is its universality of application. It must be applicable to the type of jobs for which the system was constructed.

It is best not to exceed 11 factors. It has been found that a classification system based upon 4 factors might well give the same results as one based upon 10, *if* those 4 factors are ratable, important, definitive and universal in application. It does not matter how many factors are used if those selected provide an adequate differentiation between skill levels. Sargent suggests that the following considerations be kept in mind in selecting the factors to be used: [3]

1. *Acceptability* to the parties of interest (top, middle and lower levels of management, the employees, and the union if it is involved), since the factors are the basis of the evaluations, and the objective is to establish equitable relationships which will be accepted with confidence.

2. *Applicability* to the group of jobs to be evaluated. Each factor should contribute to the evaluation of at least one job (and preferably more).

3. *Ratability*, i.e., jobs to be evaluated should carry different degrees of the factors by which they are evaluated. It is useless and confusing to use a factor which applies equally to all jobs.

4. *Distinctive nature*. Each factor should represent a separate element of job content, without overlapping another. It follows that each factor must be defined clearly.

5. *Number of factors*. It might seem that the greater this number, the greater the refinement of evaluations. This may be true, but only up to an optimum number beyond which the danger of overlapping increases and the evaluation process becomes more complex, thereby increasing time and cost of application and the likelihood of inconsistency, differences in judgment and controversy. A balance must be struck, and opinion and practice vary widely as to the optimum number. In the majority of cases, between 10 and 15 factors are used.

6. *Ease and economy of administration* tend to vary inversely with the number of factors. Reduction can be carried too far, however. Where very few (hence, very broad) factors are used, it becomes difficult to define clearly and comprehensively the ground covered by each factor and, therefore, to assure accurate and consistent application of factor scales. Resulting increases in time and cost of achieving a consensus of evaluators and management and of gaining employee and union acceptance may outweigh economies in administration.

Defining Factors and Degrees

Each factor must be clearly defined and carefully explained to the raters so that it will truly measure one and the same aspect of the total job value. If the committee has selected education as one of the factors to be rated (almost all point plans use this factor), a typical definition follows:

> This factor appraises the basic knowledge or "scholastic content" (however it may have been acquired) essential as background to learning the job. This background may have been acquired by formal education, by outside study or by on-the-job instruction at related work. The rating is expressed in terms of equivalent formal education for convenience.

In rating the job on education, *analyze the requirements of the job* regardless of the incumbent's formal education or lack of formal education.

Once the factor is defined, the number of degrees or levels within that factor must be established. Each factor must be divided into degrees which are sufficiently different so that the job rater can readily see the differences in jobs when rating them. There is no mandated number of degrees for every factor. The cardinal rule is to use only the number of degrees which are useful for differentiation. In selecting the number of degrees, it should be established that the various jobs will fall at each level. It is not necessary to have levels where no jobs fall at all. Once selecting the appropriate number of degrees, definitions must be clear and written so that the employees, supervisors and raters will understand the differences in the degrees. An example of degree definitions for the factor education follows:

First degree—knowledge of simple English grammar and arithmetic. Accuracy in checking and counting. Mental alertness and adaptability to hospital routines equivalent to four years of high school.

Second degree—knowledge of simple chemistry, biology, operation of bookkeeping or calculating machines, tabulating equipment, laboratory tools and equipment; knowledge of stenography, food preparation, etc., however acquired. Equivalent to four years of high school with specialization in science or commercial or high school plus short specialized training.

Third degree—knowledge of specialized field such as general chemistry, biology, quantitative or qualitative chemistry, nursing, accounting, drafting or statistics, or broad hospital knowledge involving complicated processes or semiprofessional services. Equivalent to four years of high school plus night, trade, extension, correspondence or state approved school in specialized training equal to two years of college.

Fourth degree—broad knowledge of general technical field such as chemistry, bacteriology, pharmacy, psychology, home economics, nursing, engineering, industrial relations, accounting, finance or business administration, however acquired. Equivalent to four years of college or university.

Fifth degree—broad knowledge of advanced and specialized field, usually equivalent to one or two years of postgraduate work.

Sixth degree—intensive knowledge of advanced and highly specialized field requiring independent research and creative work, usually equivalent to two years of postgraduate work.

In writing these degree definitions, examples should be used as much as possible. Some job evaluation manuals include pictures of the types of work which fall under a specific degree.

Determining Relative Value of Job Factors and Degrees

Once the factors are selected and defined, and further broken down into the appropriate number of degrees, it is necessary to determine the relative value of the job factor. The job evaluation committee will study the definitions of each factor. Each member will rank the factors in order of importance and distribute the share of the total to each of the factors. This process of determining the weight of each factor is usually conducted by (1) pooled judgment of the relative importance of each factor as a determinant of job content, and (2) correlation of results of these judgments with prevailing relevant pay patterns.[4]

In Exhibit 3, Point Values and Grades for Hourly Positions, 11 factors were used. The committee rated each of the factors and relative values were averaged from the committee ratings, producing a distribution of values for

Exhibit 3

POINT VALUES FOR HOURLY POSITIONS

FACTORS		DEGREES				
		1	2	3	4	5
1.	Education	15	25	40	55	70
2.	Experience	20	40	60	80	100
3.	Initiative and Ingenuity	15	25	40	55	70
4.	Physical Demand	5	10	15	20	25
5.	Mental or Visual Demand	5	10	15	20	25
6.	Responsibility for Equipment or Process	5	10	15	20	25
7.	Responsibility for Materials	5	10	15	20	25
8.	Responsibility for Safety of Others	5	10	15	20	25
9.	Responsibility for Work of Others	5	15	25	35	45
10.	Working Conditions	5	10	15	20	25
11.	Unavoidable Hazards	5	10	15	20	25

the first degree of 15 for Education, 20 for Experience, 15 for Initiative and Ingenuity and 5 each for the remaining eight factors. (Experience has demonstrated that each factor may carry a different weight.) When the relative values of the job factors are established, the committee must move toward assigning point values for each of the degrees. This can be done by arithmetic progression or geometric progression. The former method is completed by assigning values to the highest degree and the lowest degree, subtracting one from the other, and dividing the number of degrees *less one* into the difference. For example, if the lowest degree for Experience is 15 and the highest degree (the sixth degree) is 100, by dividing 5 (six degrees less one) into 85 (100 minus 15), each degree value above the first degree would be 17 points higher. Therefore, the second degree would be at a value of 32 points; the third, 49 points; the fourth, 66 points; the fifth, 83 points; and the sixth and final degree in Education would be 100 points. Using a geometric progression, one could establish by the use of logarithms the value for each degree above the first degree.

It is not unusual for the committee to assign values by a system of *value judgment,* i.e., the careful weighing and assigning of a point value, neither arithmetic nor geometric, to each degree. Some systems use a range of points for each degree, that is, for Education the first degree might be 0 to 20 points; second degree, 21 to 40 points; third degree, 41 to 60 points; fourth degree, 61 to 80 points; and fifth degree, 81 to 100 points. Such a method of assigning point values calls for precise judgment. It is almost impossible to justify the selection of 45 points as against 46 points, and although the decision as to which degree of the factor the particular job might be assigned may be quite defensible and substantiated by the description, the number of points within that degree often is a matter of unsubstantiated decision.

Advantages and Disadvantages of the Point System

The point method being a quantitative method is far more defensible than the other nonquantitative methods. The rating scale, if carefully devised and defined, permits the raters to evaluate more easily the factor against the description for the degree. In fact, agreement among various raters is usually quite close. By rating the job factor by factor, the halo effect or preconceived notions about the job based upon title or upon one aspect of the job is greatly reduced and often nullified. After rating the complete job factor by factor, the points for each factor are then totaled, thus providing a facile way of assigning jobs into various labor grades. Because of the various factors and the degrees within the factors, it is more difficult to manipulate this system than any other. Raters who gain experience in using a point method of job evaluation increase their accuracy. The evaluation of new jobs or reevaluation of jobs which have changed content appreciably is quite simple.

This method is a time-consuming method and requires precise definition of factors and degrees. The writing of these definitions requires a great deal of skill which often is not available to the institution. The assigning of point values to the factors and to the degreee is often arbitrary and in some cases difficult to defend.

The point evaluation system is the most widely used and accepted of all the job evaluation systems. It is applicable to clerical, service and maintenance jobs as well as professional jobs, each having their own set of factors weighted in accordance with the facts present in the jobs in each of those plans and divided into the necessary degrees which may differ from plan to plan.

The Factor Comparison Method.

The factor comparison method is reputed to be the method of job evaluation by which it is comparatively easy to evaluate *unlike* jobs. It is possible to use the same scale for appraising clerical, manual, creative, supervisory and executive jobs because this method does not employ specific *scales* for job measurement as does the point method. Instead *one job is compared with another.* This is essentially a ranking method; however, the ranking is done factor by factor rather than whole job by whole job. It is a quantitative system which uses analyzed judgment. Originated in 1926 by Eugene J. Benge, This method was expanded and popularized by Edward N. Hay and Samuel L. H. Burk.

There are six basic steps to the factor comparison method:

1. Determine and define the factors to be used.
2. Select and describe key jobs.
3. Rank the key jobs for each factor.
4. Apportion the money rate for each key job to the factors in the plan.
5. Establish a factor-comparison scale and add supplementary jobs.
6. Evaluate the remaining jobs by using this scale.

Benge stated that the key scale is the cardinal difference between the point system and his factor comparison method. Once it (the key scale) is established, the evaluation of jobs—like or unlike—is a simple process.

In the first step, determining and defining the factors to be used, Benge used five factors which have become standard in the construction of the factor comparison scale. The first is *mental effort* or *mental requirements.* This is defined as either the possession of and/or the active application of the following:

a. Mental traits such as intelligence, memory, reasoning, fluency, imagination and space perception.

b. General education such as grammar and arithmetic or general information as to sports, world events, etc.

c. Specialized information such as chemistry, engineering, accounting, advertising, etc.

d. Goal-setting, solutions to complex problems, analyzing cost and statistical data.

e. Writing skills, public speaking.

f. Creativity. .

The second factor is *skill*. This is defined as:

a. Facility in muscular coordination as in operating machines, repetitive movements, careful coordinations, dexterity assembling, sorting, etc.

b. Specific job "know-how" necessary to the muscular coordination only, acquired by performance of the work and not to be confused with general education or specialized information. It is very largely training in the interpretation of sensory impressions.

The third factor is *physical effort* or *physical requirements*. This is defined as:

a. Physical effort such as sitting, standing, walking, climbing, pulling, lifting. Both the amount exercised and the degree of the continuity should be taken into account.

b. Physical status such as age, height, weight, sex, strength and eyesight.

The fourth factor is *responsibilities*. This is defined as responsibilities for:

a. Raw materials, processed materials, tools, equipment and property.

b. Money or negotiable securities.

c. Profits or loss, savings or methods improvement.

d. Public contact.

e. Records.

f. Supervision. Under supervision, the rater is asked to evaluate the complexity of supervision given to subordinates. The number of subordinates in the secondary position. Responsibility for planning, directing, coordinating. Also the degree of supervision received rather than given, as above.

The fifth and last factor is *working conditions*. This is defined as:

a. Environmental influences such as atmosphere, ventilation, illumination, noise, congestion.

b. Hazards.

c. Hours.

If an institution desires to construct its own factor comparison job evaluation system, it is not advisable to use more than seven factors. The factors selected must be defined clearly to ensure uniform interpretation by the rating committee.

The second step is to select key jobs which are indeed the core of the rating scale upon which other jobs will be rated. A key job representing a cross-section of all jobs should be selected for each of the pay levels. The most important element is that current pay rates for the job must be considered fair in relation to other jobs in the *hospital* or *home* and the *community*. The key jobs should be stable and well-defined. Job specifications should be written in terms of the factors used in this scale; the job specification would include a section for mental requirements, skill, physical requirements, responsibilities and working conditions. It is advisable to use from 24 to 30 key jobs in constructing the scale. A cross-section of jobs from each department, or from the key departments, should be chosen with specific care to select such jobs which are recognized to be high, medium and low in worth. When the key jobs have been selected, copies of the job descriptions and job specifications for each of the jobs are to be distributed to members of the ranking committee.

The third step is ranking the key jobs under each factor. Since the factor comparison method is essentially a ranking method, evaluators must consider all the key jobs one factor at a time. Pooled judgment is an outstanding characteristic of factor comparison. It is customary to have 4 to 10 evaluators, each of whom expresses his judgment individually in writing about the ranking of each key job, factor by factor. The evaluators keeping the job specification and job description in mind approach the first factor, mental efforts and make a judgment as to which key job requires the least and the greatest amount of this factor. This judgment may be marked on a card. The committee then compares their rankings, and discrepancies are discussed at this point. It may well occur that the rankings of one or two persons are so atypical that they should be discarded in coming up with the average ranking. This method is similar to the method used in judging Olympic diving performances, where the scores of the judges with the highest score and the lowest score are disregarded in arriving at the total score. Clearing up the discrepancies which may well be caused by a lack of complete knowledge of the job, all the rankings are averaged for that factor (see Exhibit 4).

The next step is probably one of the most difficult: apportioning the money rate for each key job to the factors in the plan. The evaluators must consider each job in turn and express their opinions as to the percentage of

Exhibit 4

RANKS ASSIGNED TO KEY JOBS

JOB	Mental Effort					Skill					Physical Requirements					Responsibility					Working Conditions				
	Ranker A	B	C	D	Ave.	Ranker A	B	C	D	Ave.	Ranker A	B	C	D	Ave.	Ranker A	B	C	D	Ave.	Ranker A	B	C	D	Ave.
Food Preparer	9	10	10	10	10	7	9	8	7	8	7	6	6	6	6	9	10	9	9	9	7	7	6	7	7
Laundry Worker	10	9	9	9	9	6	8	6	6	6	3	3	3	4	3	8	9	7	8	8	2	2	2	2	2
Nurses Aide	6	8	6	6	6	4	5	5	5	5	8	9	7	8	8	7	8	6	7	7	8	8	9	8	9
Messenger	11	11	12	11	11	12	12	12	12	12	5	4	4	3	4	11	7	11	11	10	10	9	10	10	10
Medical Rec. Clk.	7	7	8	8	8	8	6	7	8	7	4	5	5	5	5	10	11	10	10	11	6	5	7	9	6
Lab. Tech.	3	2	3	3	3	1	1	2	1	1	9	8	9	9	9	3	2	2	2	2	9	10	8	5	8
Surgical Tech.	4	5	4	4	4	2	2	1	3	2	10	10	11	10	10	6	5	8	6	6	1	1	1	1	1
Pharmacist	1	1	1	1	1	5	3	4	4	4	11	11	10	11	11	1	1	1	1	1	11	12	11	11	11
Porter	12	12	11	12	12	10	11	11	11	11	1	2	2	2	2	12	12	12	12	12	5	6	5	6	5
Storekeeper	8	6	7	7	7	9	10	10	10	10	2	1	1	1	1	4	4	4	4	4	3	4	3	3	3
Cook	5	4	5	5	5	3	4	3	2	3	6	7	8	7	7	5	6	5	5	5	4	3	4	4	4
Dietitian	2	3	2	2	2	11	7	9	9	9	12	12	12	12	12	2	3	3	3	3	12	11	12	12	12

the salary presently paid for that job which is judged to be paid for each of the five factors. For example, if a nurses' aide is paid $4 an hour, a judgment must be made as to what part of that total $4 is paid for mental efforts, skill, physical efforts, responsibilities and working conditions. Each evaluator is asked to determine how much of the total rate for the job is paid for each of the five factors. The going rate for the key job is used. If more than one person occupies a key job, which is quite likely, the average rate paid for that group is used as the going rate for the job. Once this is determined, the scale is then set up on the basis of units or, in most cases, the basis of money.

Finally the fifth step, the heart of the factor comparison method, is the establishment of the factor comparison scale. The scale has five horizontal columns, one for each factor. Vertical columns designate a cents-per-hour scale. Each key job is placed in position on the scale for each of the factors. For example, the committee has determined that the laundry worker's job is broken down as follows: mental effort, 20 percent; skill, 40 percent; physical effort, 10 percent; responsibilities, 10 percent; working conditions, 20 percent. The laundry worker is paid a going rate of $3.50 per hour. That position would then be placed alongside the $.70 mark on the vertical scale in the mental effort column; alongside the $1.40 mark in the skill column; alongside the $.35 mark in both the physical effort column and the responsibilities column; and finally, alongside the $.70 mark in the working conditions column. The same method would be used to place the other key jobs at various levels in the various factors (see Exhibit 5).

The remaining jobs are handled by using the following three-step method. First, the committee studies the specifications factor by factor. Then each factor is judged against jobs that are currently on the rating scale. One consideration, for example, is whether the mental effort of the job to be evaluated is greater or less than that for a specific job already placed on the factor comparison scale. Finally, as the job is evaluated, it can be entered upon the scale.

Assumptions under the Factor Comparison Method

Benge made numerous assumptions about the factor comparison method which make this method one of the strongest of the job evaluation systems:

1. The factor comparison scale should be expressed in monetary units.

2. The factors used should not exceed seven.

3. Job specifications are necessary and should be written in terms of the factors to be used on the scale.

4. There should be no upper limit to the amount of money allowable for a given factor.

5. Each job factor should be compared with the same factor in another job, thus employing job-to-job comparison rather than job-to-predetermined scale comparison.

6. Pooled judgment on the basis of repeated judgments of competent evaluators should be used in obtaining final figures.

Advantages and Disadvantages of the Factor Comparison Method

This method is a difficult plan to implement because the selection of the key jobs is the core of a successful program, and these jobs must have duties that are clearly defined and rates that are not subject to controversy. Once the scale is constructed, the evaluation of the remaining jobs can be simply and expertly completed. One overriding advantage of the factor comparison method is that the scales are open-ended and the scale for any factor may be extended upward or downward at any time.[5]

Exhibit 5

UNITS	MENTAL REQUIREMENTS	SKILL REQUIREMENTS	PHYSICAL REQUIREMENTS	RESPONSIBILITY	WORKING CONDITIONS	UNITS
130						130
129						129
128						128
127		Lab. Tech.				127
126						126
125						125
124						124
123		Surg. Tech.				123
122						122
121						121
120						120
119						119
118	Pharmacist					118
117						117
116						116
115						115
114				Pharmacist		114
113						113
112	Dietician					112
111						111
∿	∿	∿	∿	∿	∿	∿
103	Lab. Tech.					103
102						102
101						101
100						100
∿	∿	∿	∿	∿	∿	∿
49						49
48			Storekeeper			48
47					Surg. Tech.	47
46	Cook					46
45	Med. Records Clk.		Porter	Lab. Tech.	Storekeeper	45
44						44
43						43
42			Surg. Tech.			42
41						41
40					Porter	40
39						39
38	Porter	Cook				38
37			Cook	Med. Records Clk.		37
36						36
35			Lab. Tech.			35
34						34
33				Porter	Cook	33
32						32
31						31
30						30
29		Med. Records Clk.			Messenger	29
28						28
27						27
26						26
25						25
24		Porter				24
23						23
22						22
21			Pharmacist			21
20					Dietician	20
19						19
18						18
17						17
16						16
15					Pharmacist	15
14						14
13						13
12						12
∿	∿	∿	∿	∿	∿	∿
5						5
4						4
3						3
2						2
1						1

Job Evaluation Manuals

The job evaluation manual is developed in the initial stages of the program to aid the raters and to obtain the understanding of supervisors and employees. Each factor has an overall explanation and each degree has a definitive description. The manual will outline the methods for evaluating the jobs and will contain, wherever possible, illustrations of bench-mark jobs for each of the factors and for each of the degrees or levels. Addendum A to this chapter is from a job evaluation manual and includes a description of factors and degrees of rating *hourly* positions; bench-mark jobs for hourly position factors and degrees; and point values and grades for hourly positions. This addendum is based on a point method of job evaluation.[6]

Wage and Salary Administration

A sound wage and salary administration program is essential to the success of any individual enterprise; its importance is now widely recognized.[7]

Enlightened management today is, above all, responsible management. It recognizes the obligations inherent in the function of leadership. Among the most prominent of these obligations is that of compensating employees in both financial and nonfinancial terms for their vital contribution to the success of the enterprise.[8]

With salaries constituting between 60 and 70 percent of the budget of a health service institution, it becomes necessary for the administration to implement sound controls over wages and salaries. Most institutions establish their compensation objectives in advance of pricing and controlling salaries. The following is an example of one institution's compensation policy:

1. Pay employees at rates equal to or better than rates for positions requiring comparable skill, effort and responsibility in the community.

2. Establish and maintain fair wage differentials between jobs in all departments in terms of the value of each job to the institution.

3. Pay all employees in accordance with all applicable federal and state legislation or regulations as to wages, hours and other conditions of work.

4. Follow the principle of equal pay for equal work assignments.

5. Recognize and reward employees based on their individual ability, outstanding performance and length of service within the rate range established for the job occupied.

It is obvious that the key to a successful wage and salary program is the establishment of fair wage standards.

Constructing a Wage Curve: The Wage Survey

Job pricing is the cornerstone of wage and salary administration. Constructing a wage structure may indeed be the most difficult task confronting the individuals delegated the responsibility for implementing a sound wage and salary program. Rates of pay for each job must be obtained either by securing the comparative rates paid in the local community or in the general health services industry and developing a wage curve based upon a quantitative value and those rates obtained from the community or industry, or by devising a wage curve based upon the institution's present rates and comparing this curve with the community rates.

The wage curve is a graphic presentation which displays the relationship between the quantitative value as depicted by the points in a point system or evaluated rates of the factor-comparison method and some wage standard. The wage standard may develop from any one of the following:

1. The present rates paid by the institution.
2. Community rates for certain key jobs.
3. Rates established by collective bargaining. Many systems establish a wage curve based upon the evaluated point values and the institution's current rates. The primary assumption in this method is that the institution's current rates, except for a limited amount of inequities, are sound. It is a far more defensible approach to incorporate in juxtaposition to a wage curve based upon the institution's present rates, a wage curve based upon going community rates. By presenting these two wage curves, a visual comparison is made possible, and more often than not *the wage curve line finally developed is a compromise between the two.*

It is essential in sound wage determination and basic to a sound wage and salary program that the institution pay competitive wages. Therefore, the wage survey is at the core of institution job pricing. The wage survey seeks to identify comparative rates for comparable jobs in a particular labor market such as the locality in which the health service institution is situated or in the health service industry in general. There are four specific comparisons which may be made between one institution's rates and the rates paid by other institutions in the survey. These are: hiring rates, base rates, averaged earned rates and additions to income.

The hiring rate is not always the base rate for the job since it is often dependent upon market pressures including shortages of key skills. The average earned rate gives a clear indication of increases based on seniority and merit. Under the additions-to-income comparison, recognition of the value of fringe benefits is essential for any valid comparison.

Conducting a wage survey is not a simple matter. There are three methods commonly used to obtain information by conducting a wage survey:

1. A job title survey.
2. A job description survey.
3. A job evaluation survey.

The *job title survey* is usually conducted by telephone or letter. It is an informal method and often inaccurate because of the limited details provided as to the specifications of the jobs. Although in some matters "a rose is a rose is a rose," in conducting wage surveys, one often finds that a nurse's aide is not a nurse's aide is not a nurse's aide. Job titles may be similar and yet employees with such titles may have different duties at different institutions. A proper comparison of wages cannot be made unless the exact details of the jobs being compared are available from the job description.

The *job description survey* can be conducted either by mail or by personal interview. Participating institutions are asked to identify the wage rates for the jobs in their organization which have duties similar to those in the job descriptions provided. The survey is often limited to selected "key jobs" ranging from the lowest to the highest grade. In such a survey the process of selecting key jobs is a critical one. It is most important that a fair sample of jobs in the organization be the decisive factor in choosing those jobs to be surveyed. A job description of each key job is forwarded to the participating institutions (see Exhibit 6, page 85). This reduces the inaccuracies and facilitates the comparisons. The selection of jobs to be priced deserves further comment. Emphasis must be placed on representative jobs—those around which a number of other jobs can be priced. The key jobs, or representative ones, should be easy to identify and define, well-known and comparable to those in other institutions included in the survey. In addition, such jobs should be filled by a large group of employees.

The *job evaluation survey* is limited to institutions using the same job evaluation method so that the point value for each job in the survey can be equated to a job of equal value in the other institutions. This often is not possible in the health services industry since few institutions use similar job evaluation methods. It has been successfully and widely used in the metal trades and in the electrical industry.

The task of conducting the survey should be assigned to the wage and salary division of the personnel department. The individual who is specifically assigned to conduct the survey should have expert knowledge of wage payment methods and wage and salary administration. When the survey information has been obtained, a tabulation must be completed. This tabulation includes the posting of wage rates for each specific key job. It is useful to calculate the median rate for each of those jobs. There are many uses of the survey information [9]

1. To establish hiring rates which will attract new employees.

2. As a basis for rate changes to prevent abnormal turnover due to inadequacy of compensation and also to minimize "labor pirating."

Exhibit 6

Job Description Survey

MESSENGER

Runs errands and performs simple clerical duties.
Picks up and sorts letters, messages, packages,
records, interoffice memoranda, and other items,
and delivers them to various offices and departments.
Runs errands for staff, making trips to and from
outside establishments to deliver and obtain messages
and small articles. May mail outgoing letters and
packages, operate automatic stamping machine, weigh
and stamp heavy mail, and keep records of envelopes
and stamps in stock. Performs a variety of related
tasks, such as cleaning office machines, assisting in
stockroom, and filing material where little knowledge
of subject matter is required.

Pay Rate: Minimum_____   Maximum_____
             Raise Increments_____

Pay rate shown (check one):
     Hourly_____ Daily_____ Weekly_____
     Bi-weekly____ Semi-monthly____ Monthly____

Is overtime paid?   Yes_____   No_____

If overtime is paid, check rate paid for work in excess
of 40-hour week:
        1____ 1.5____ 2____ 2.5____ Other(signify)___

Schedule:
     Hours/shift____Hours/week____Days/week_____
     Split shift:Yes___ No___ Weekends:Yes___ No__

Is this job part of any bargaining union?   _____
     If so, what union?   _____

Number of employees in this job: _____

3. To keep abreast of pay rate trends which have a direct bearing on the cost of services rendered.

4. To enable an institution to minimize employee dissatisfaction with compensation rates though such dissatisfaction does not cause many resignations.

5. To implement institutional policy which emphasizes that the institution pays community rates or better.

6. To determine the extent of the employee benefits and services offered in addition to direct pay rates.

Pricing the Jobs

Armed with information on the base rate, the median rate and the going rate (the rate which a good, average employee will reach after he learns his job well), the person in charge makes a comparison with the current rates paid at his institution. Next he makes a base rate comparison. In order to complete this comparison, an analysis of the institution's payroll must be conducted. Tabulation of the base rates of each employee in each key job must be made. Finally, a median rate for each key job must be established. A graph is then completed. It will have labor grades or evaluated point values along the abscissa and current money rates along (up) the ordinate. The salaries for key jobs presently in effect at the institution are plotted. The current wage curve is drawn from those rates. A similar procedure is followed for the survey rates for participating hospitals (see Exhibit 7, next page).

Otis and Leukart list the following steps in constructing the wage survey:[10]

1. Obtain present rates (going rates) being paid for key jobs. Use either average or median rate. The median rate is better if there are extreme rates in the sample (a very low rate or a very high rate). Establish one rate for the key job.

2. Obtain evaluated point value for key jobs.

3. Position each key job on chart by locating going rate on vertical and point value on horizontal.

4. Trend line is then drawn freehand, either straight or curved or calculated on the basis of least squares method.

Before undertaking the establishment of a sound wage and salary administration program, the personnel department must be apprised of the institution's philosophy, specifically its wage policy. Will the institution undertake to establish a wage program which is competitive with the going rates in the community and the industry? This is the key question. With the

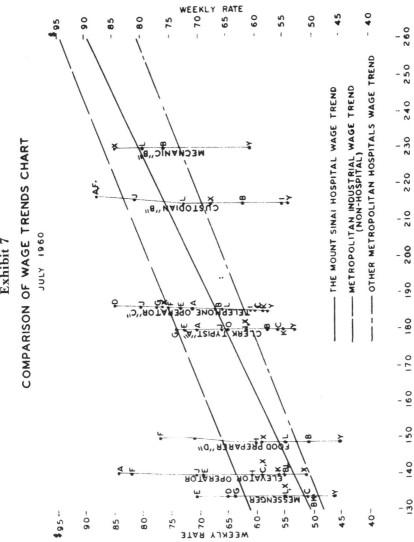

Exhibit 7

COMPARISON OF WAGE TRENDS CHART

JULY 1960

institution's policy as a guideline, the wage and salary administrator can then determine which adjustments must be made in the institution's wage curve to bring it into line with that of the community or the industry.

Rate Ranges

The trend line is the salient point to pricing the jobs. Once this trend line is established, labor grades can be developed which provide for movement from minimum to maximum rate for the job. There are two other methods of wage payments. The first is individual rates wherein each job is priced individually, and there are as many rates as there are individual jobs. Where there are many jobs, it is a cumbersome task for the personnel department to deal with such individual rates. This method should be discouraged. The second method is the single rate method where jobs are assigned to a number of classes and all jobs falling in a particular class are given the same wage. This type of wage rate schedule allows no range in salary and requires the payment of the same wage to each individual employee on the job or in the job class. This is a method favored by unions who prefer movement of employee salaries based upon collective bargaining. Once negotiating this type of wage structure in a union contract, the institution should resist additional increases through step structures which provide not only the across-the-board increase, but also a "seniority" increase.

The rate range structure is widely used in the administration of non-unionized positions. Three decisions must be made in establishing a rate range: (1) the width of the grade, (2) the spread between the minimum and maximum rates of the range, and (3) the extent of overlap of one range and the next higher range.[11] The width of the range has to do with the number of jobs which will fall into a single grade. If the institution is using a point method, this decision must be determined on the point value of the jobs. If many jobs are put in one grade and they have a wide range in their point value, this grade will be, perforce, a very wide one. One of the cardinal factors in establishing a cutoff as to the width of the grade is the natural progression of jobs. For example, the laboratory technician may have three classifications based upon experience and complexity of work. In the establishment of grades, it behooves the wage and salary administrator to have Laboratory Technician A in a higher grade than Laboratory Technician B, and Laboratory Technician B in a higher grade than Laboratory Technician C. This may well determine the width of a grade and which jobs are to be included in which grades. The cutoff is often made simpler by the determination of a point cutoff (see Exhibit 8, next page).

Exhibit 8

Key to Grades for Salary Positions

Grade	Point Range
11	150 and under
10	151-190
9	191-230
8	231-270
7	271-310
6	311-350
5	351-390
4	391-430
3	431-470
2	471-510
1	511-550

A chart of progression (see Exhibit 9, next page) is useful to examine the appropriateness of grades.

It is usually possible to upgrade an employee more easily if provision is based upon an extremely fine difference in difficulty levels between jobs. For example, a job in one grade is probably a shade less difficult than a job on the next higher grade. If an institution decides to have many grades, it will result in a very narrow wage range for each grade or a very wide overlap in grades. If you provide fewer labor grades, a wider range develops. This allows the institution to give many merit increases and reward seniority within a labor grade. Of course, wide ranges have the concomitant over-lapping of grades which will cause some of the workers in a lower grade to earn more than some of the workers in a higher grade. The justification for such overlap is that a seasoned employee in a lower grade can easily be worth more than a beginner in a higher grade. Such an overlap also provides a desirable flexibility for the transfer of employees from a lower labor grade to a higher one without large increases. One serious disadvantage of many labor grades is that they decrease distinguishable differences in difficulty level between grades. Today's trend is toward providing as few labor grades as possible. This has several advantages. The chances of having adjacent labor grades which are not distinguishably different is greatly reduced. A wider range can be assigned each class without having a large overlap in wages which provides for more opportunity for merit rating and movement

Exhibit 9

CHART OF PROGRESSION

	FOOD SERVICES (000–099)	BUILDING SERVICES (100–199)	NURSING SERVICES (200–299)	TECHNICAL (300–499)	CLERICAL (500–599)	ADMINISTRATIVE (600–899)
1S						
2S	FOOD SUPERVISOR (MANAGER) A					
3S				PHARMACIST (CHIEF) A		
4S			NURSE A			
1H						
5S		LAUNDRY SUPERVISOR (MANAGER) A		PHARMACIST B		PERSONNEL ADMINISTRATOR
2H						
3H						
6S	DIETITIAN A / FOOD PREPARER A	FOREMAN A	NURSE B	PHARMACIST C / LABORATORY SUPERVISOR A	SECRETARY A	ASSISTANT PURCHASING AGENT
4H						
7S	DIETITIAN B	FOREMAN B	NURSE C	PHARMACIST D / LABORATORY SUPERVISOR B	SECRETARY B	TELEPHONE OPERATOR (CHIEF) A / CUSTODIAN (CHIEF OFFICER) A / TRAFFIC AND INFORMATION SUPERVISOR A
5H		MECHANIC A				
6H				LABORATORY TECHNICIAN A		
8S	FOOD SUPERVISOR B / FOOD PREPARER B / DIETITIAN C	FOREMAN C	NURSE D	LABORATORY SUPERVISOR C	REGISTRAR A	PRINTER A
7H		MECHANIC B		LABORATORY TECHNICIAN B		
9S		LAUNDRY WORKER			SECRETARY C / MEDICAL OFFICE ASSISTANT	
8H	FOOD PREPARER C	MECHANIC C	NURSE (PRACTICAL) E		STENOGRAPHER	STOREROOM ATTENDANT A / TELEPHONE OPERATOR B
9H		MECHANIC D / MAINTENANCE A / LAUNDRY WORKER A	NURSE AUXILIARY A		REGISTRAR B / CLERK-TYPIST A	TELEPHONE OPERATOR C & STOREROOM ATTENDANT B / CUSTODIAN B
10S	FOOD SUPERVISOR C					HOUSEMOTHER / TRAFFIC AND INFORMATION SUPERVISOR B
10H		LAUNDRY WORKER B / MAINTENANCE B		LABORATORY TECHNICIAN C		PRINTER B / PROJECTIONIST / SALESMAN
11S	FOOD SUPERVISOR D					
11H	DIETITIAN (WORKER) D / FOOD PREPARER D	MECHANIC / MAINTENANCE C / LAUNDRY WORKER C	NURSE AUXILIARY B / NURSE AUXILIARY C	PHARMACIST (NON-PROF) E / LABORATORY TECHNICIAN	REGISTRAR C / CLERK-TYPIST B / CLERK	ELEVATOR OPERATOR / MESSENGER / CUSTODIAN C / ATTENDANT

within a range. Usually 10 to 12 labor grades are used, but plans range from 8 to 16 labor grades. As to overlapping, the trend is to reduce the overlap as much as possible. This will obviate the problem of an individual in a higher labor class receiving less money than one in a lower labor class.

The spread between the minimum and maximum rates of the range is often determined by the following factors: (1) frequency of salary reviews, (2) the learning time, and (3) proper incentive. Some plans use a constant spread throughout each grade. Others use variable spreads (less of a spread for low rated jobs; more of a spread for higher rated jobs). Less than a 20 percent spread does not provide sufficient incentive. It is more common to find a spread of 35 percent. Such a spread is in most cases sufficient for nonexempt positions, but a 50 percent spread is usually better for exempt jobs.[12] The use of a constant dollar limit on the spread is inadvisable since it tends to telescope the labor grade system and penalize jobs in the higher labor grades. The constant percentage limit method provides for the same percentage spread within each range. This, of course, results in unnecessary and unmanageable overlap. A variable percentage limit method can overcome this problem. Here a larger percentage spread is used in upper grades than in lower grades.

The third consideration is the extent of overlap. Will the maximum of a lower labor grade be the same as the minimum of the next higher labor grade? The provision for overlapping grades is not unusual where the next higher labor grade starts at a point somewhere between the midpoint and the maximum of the lower labor grade.

Establishing a labor grade structure that meets a particular institution's needs will involve experimentation to ensure:

1. Proper incentive within a grade by establishing an inadequate spread.

2. Appropriate differentials between grades by holding the overlap to a fair percentage.

Once the trend line is established, labor grades can be developed which provide movement from minimum to maximum. Points on the trend line may be used as the midpoint for each labor grade. The usual practice is to establish a rate range with a spread from minimum to maximum of 20 to 40 percent. Ranges in most plans will overlap each other. A differential, *the difference between the minimum of a labor grade and the minimum of the next higher labor grade,* of 9 to 15 percent is usual.

Employee Pay Rates

Once the labor grade structure is developed, a determination of each employee's pay rate follows. It may be useful to evaluate the performance of each employee to determine which position he will take in a newly established rate range. Specific rates for each step within the rate range are necessary to provide maximum control over movement within that range. Progression from the minimum to the maximum in a labor grade may be either automatic or based on merit. The automatic method provides for a period in which the pay rate is increased from minimum to maximum based on seniority within the labor grade. This method is favored by labor unions. Progressing through the rate range on the basis of merit offers complete flexibility within a range. The worker can be placed at any point within the rate range on the basis of job effectiveness as compared with that of other employees in a similar classification. This offers maximum incentive for employees to improve their efficiency. A compromise would incorporate both merit and automatic progression. An employee would automatically progress from the minimum to the midpoint of the range on the basis of seniority, moving through the steps up to the midpoint on specific anniversary dates. Once reaching the midpoint of the range, the employee's movement from that point to the maximum would be based upon merit.

Coding of Jobs

When the salary structure has been established and each employee's rate determined, a uniform and consistent administration must be assured. In order to do this, a well-managed record system should be instituted.

The first step in such a system is the coding of jobs. A simple eight-digit code is commonly used. The first three digits of the code denote the department. The next two digits are used for position title or function. The sixth digit is class and the last two digits are the position number. For example, let us look at the laundry department of the hospital. It had been determined that there are three levels of laundry workers. Laundry Worker C includes people who are responsible for sorting, folding, packing, collecting and feeding. The next highest is Laundry Worker B, which includes the tumbler, lead seamstress, lead flatwork operator, lead packer and lead collector. The highest level of laundry worker is Laundry Worker A, who is the washer. The department number for the laundry is 321, which would be the first three digits of the code. Laundry Worker is 13, the fourth and fifth digits of the code. Laundry Worker A would have a 1 as the sixth digit of the code. The last two digits, which denote the position number, reflect each authorized position in a table of organization within each master job classification, so that if there are ten Laundry Worker A's they would be numbered from 01 to 10. Therefore, Laundry Worker A would have as his eight-digit code, 321-131-01. Laundry Worker B would be 321-132-01. Laundry Worker C would be 321-133-01. If there were a second Laundry Worker C, his code would be 321-133-02.

Responsibility for the Wage and Salary Policies

It is important that the institution develop a clear policy covering wage and salary administration including the responsibilities for such policies. One institution outlines such responsibilities as follows.

1. It is the responsibility of the personnel director to:

a. establish wage objectives and approve wage and salary policies;

b. coordinate the activities involved in handling of wage matters and evaluate performances against these objectives; and

c. provide an adequately trained wage and salary administration staff to provide necessary technical assistance to the line, prepare and update job descriptions and perform job analysis and evaluations.

Another organization states its policies regarding wage and salary administration as follows.

1. The personnel director is the executive director's designated representative for the administration of programs to implement approved wage and salary objectives and policies. He or she is responsible for:

a. ensuring that the approved salary and wage administration policies, programs and procedures are administered to meet the institution's requirements;

b. recommending changes in wage and salary objectives and policies required by changed conditions or as approved by the board of trustees.

c. developing institution-wide compensation evaluation and merit rating plans and procedures;

d. classifying all jobs into their appropriate job classification and grade according to their functional requirements;

e. establishing and approving the rate of compensation each employee is to receive for the performance of work on either an hourly or salary basis;

f. approving all employee transfers, promotions, demotions, merit increases or other changes that may affect pay;

g. notifying the comptroller's office of each employee's rate or change in rate;

h. approving and preparing job specifications, rates and "slotting" new positions in the institution after submission by the appropriate administrator prior to the organizational establishment of the job;

i. establishing and performing periodic checks to ascertain and assure that all employees are properly classified according to the duties they perform;

j. conducting periodic wage and salary surveys necessary for the maintenance of equitable ongoing rates for positions in the institution;

k. administering the merit rating plan and policies to ensure accurate and just ratings;

l. conducting periodic audits of the wage and salary administration program, wage objectives and policies, organization structure for salary administration, merit rating plan, wage practices and salary administration.

Wage and Salary Forms

The design of appropriate forms is a cardinal consideration in developing necessary controls over wages and salaries.

The individual form should normally be designed around the administrative system rather than the other way around. It has neither purpose nor meaning in itself except in terms of the context of processes which accompany its preparation and completion. The forms employed in the personnel department, then, should be custom designed to fit the specific situation at hand. Some questions which should normally be asked when designing such forms are as follows:

1. How many people need either to review the form or to verify its contents before it becomes an official document of the business? The answers to this question may take a number of directions as far as designing the form is concerned. For instance, if only a few people need know that an action has occurred, a manifold form which can be completed, torn apart, and sent in several directions at once may be quite satisfactory. If, on the other hand, certain authenticating signatures are required before the form becomes an official document of the business, it may be sufficient to design a single-page form with a set of locations for required signatures. In some cases, a combination of both the manifold and the required signature boxes may be the best approach.

2. What are the requirements and constraints related to storing the document? Is there any particular file size which must be adhered to, as, for instance 5 by 8 in. or 8½ by 11 in. file folders? Does all data related to a document have to be contained in one 8½ by 11 in. sheet in order to reduce it to storage in, say, a microfilm type of form? Is the form itself designed for direct access, as with certain records of the Cardex or Visadex type, where one edge is displayed for screening or scanning purposes? How much emphasis must be placed upon producing a record which can be preserved for long periods at low expense?

3. Who is going to be responsible for completing the form? If a trained

personnel clerk will be doing the job, it is quite possible to leave the form in a much more complex state than if any random employee has to complete it. Application blanks, for instance, need to have highly simplified formats which guide the candidate step by step through the process of supplying the data needed. They must make it easy for him to provide that data in the form wanted and must avoid the appearance of overcomplexity or invasion of the individual's privacy. Addition-to-payroll forms, on the other hand—particularly those which are completed by trained clerks who know how to obtain a high degree of rapport with the people supplying them with needed information—may be very complex in design and may ask for data in greater detail in sensitive areas without creating any particular problems. If the form is designed for completion by an individual manager or his secretary, it must not be so complex that it either discourages proper completion or requires excessive training time of the people who are to complete it. If training is required, as, for instance, for secretaries of managers who are responsible for inputting these forms, arrangements must be made for continual training so as to provide the necessary instruction to newly appointed secretaries to such managers.

4. When data must be transferred from the original form to a secondary storage source, the manner in which the data is originally captured should be optimized for purposes of accurate and efficient transferral. To the greatest degree possible, the data should be entered in a fashion which permits direct extraction from the original document at absolute minimum effort so as to assure quick, accurate transcription and verification of the data.

5. New forms should always be pretested on the employees, applicants, and clerical personnel who will be using them. If necessary, formal tests should be conducted to determine which of several available formats is easiest to use from everyone's point of view. Too many forms are merely concocted on the spur of the moment to meet an assumed need without any reference to the people who will have to live with them after they have been printed up.

6. The purposes and objectives which the data is to serve should be specifically and explicitly defined so that determination can be made of whether the form is meeting real data needs or not.[13]

A *requisition form* for personnel is the cornerstone of the wage and salary administration system. It is used to establish a new position, to ensure appropriate administrative approval concerning the legitimacy of the need, to aid in recruitment and to initiate payroll action. It is also used for personnel replacements. The requisition form should contain provisions for documentation of special hiring arrangements and comments about future salary reviews. Exhibit 10 (see page 96) is an example of such a form. It is a five-copy set. The originating department keeps one copy before for-

Exhibit 10

LAURICT PRINTING CO., INC., 342 WEST 14TH STREET, NEW YORK 14, N. Y. OR 5-2250

THE MOUNT SINAI HOSPITAL
PERSONNEL REQUISITION

51033 1P

RECEIVED BY PERSONNEL

REQUISITION NUMBER
20272

1. DATE PREPARED

2. SIGNATURE OF ORIGINATOR

3. DEPARTMENT

6. JOB CLASSIFICATION

7. GRADE

8. POSITION OR FUNCTIONAL TITLE

9. POSITION #

4. EMPLOYMENT REQUISITION - COMPLETE THIS SECTION IF REQUEST IS TO FILL A POSITION

☐ TO FILL NEW POSITION (COMPLETE SECTION 5)

☐ REPLACEMENT FOR   LAST NAME   FIRST NAME   EMPLOYEE #

{ ☐ L.O.A. RELIEF FOR   LAST NAME   FIRST NAME   EMPLOYEE #

☐ TERMINATED ON ____ DATE ____ TO ____ DEPT. ____ POSITION #

☐ TRANSFERRED ON ____ DATE ____ TO ____ DEPT.

☐ IS ON L.O.A. FROM ____ DATE ____ TO ____ DATE ____ TO BE REFERRED FOR FINAL INTERVIEW BY:

☐ MALE   APPLICANTS PREFERRED
☐ FEMALE

APPROPRIATE DEPARTMENT MEMBER   EXTENSION

NOTE: AN APPLICANT WILL NOT BE PUT ON PAYROLL NOR WILL HE BE RECOGNIZED AS AN EMPLOYEE UNLESS HE IS FIRST PROCESSED AND THEN HIS EMPLOYMENT IS CONFIRMED WITH A PERSONNEL DIRECTLY AFTER HE HAS STARTED WORK.

10. HOURS OF WORK   MON. TUES. WED. THUR. FRI. SAT. SUN. VARIABLE
    ☐ ☐ ☐ ☐ ☐ ☐ ☐ ☐

HRS./WK. FROM ____ AM ____ TO ____ AM
                        PM   PM

11. HIRING SALARY RANGE

FROM $ ____   (HIRING RATE, JOB RATE, OR OTHER ESTABLISHED MINIMUM SALARY FOR THIS POSITION.)

TO $ ____   (MAXIMUM OFFERING SALARY CONSISTENT WITH CURRENT DEPARTMENTAL SALARIES AND WITHIN LIMITS OF AVAILABLE FUNDS.)

12. SALARY SOURCE

☐ 100% BUDGETARY ☐ 100% FUND #

____ % BUDGETARY ____ % FUND #

PROJECT # ____ APPROVAL DATE ____

FUNDS APPROVED FROM ____ TO ____

NOTED BY
FUND ACCOUNTANT ____ DATE ____

5. POSITION REQUISITION — COMPLETE THIS SECTION AND OBTAIN APPROPRIATE AUTHORIZATIONS IF REQUEST IS TO ESTABLISH NEW POSITION:

POSITION SHOULD BE:

☐ PERMANENT (NAP)

{ ☐ TEMPORARY (TAP) FROM ____ TO ____ DATE

☐ VACATION RELIEF (VRP) ____ DATE

{ ☐ FULL TIME

☐ PART TIME (____ HRS./WK.)   ESTIMATED SALARY COST FOR NEW POSITION: $ ____

EXPLAIN NEED FOR NEW POSITION; ATTACH SUPPORTING DATA IF NECESSARY:

13. DUTIES, RESPONSIBILITIES, EDUCATION, EXPERIENCE, LICENSES, AND SPECIAL QUALIFICATIONS FOR POSITION (THIS SECTION NEED NOT BE COMPLETED IF PERSONNEL HAS AN APPROVED POSITION DESCRIPTION OR IF FUNCTION IS OBVIOUS FROM TITLE):

ATTACH A COMPLETED JOB INFORMATION FORM, OR COMPLETE SEC. 13 IF POSITION CAN BE DESCRIBED BRIEFLY.

SUGGESTED POSITION TITLE:

PROPOSED JOB CLASSIFICATION:

CLASSIFICATION APPROVED BY
WAGE & SALARY ADMINISTRATOR _____ DATE _____

NEW POSITION APPROVED BY
ASST. DIRECTOR (FUND ACCT. FOR FUNDED POS.) _____ DATE _____

NEW POSITION AUTHORIZED BY
DIRECTOR OR ASSOC. DIRECTOR _____ DATE _____

14. SPECIAL EMPLOYMENT OR SALARY ARRANGEMENTS

APPROPRIATE APPROVAL _____ DATE _____

EMPLOYMENT INFORMATION AND PAYROLL ACTION

TO BE COMPLETED BY PERSONNEL DEPARTMENT

DO NOT WRITE BELOW THIS LINE

| 15. NAME | M ☐ F ☐ | 16. EMPLOYEE # | 17. SOCIAL SECURITY # | 18. BIRTH DATE | 19. MARITAL STATUS | 20. CITIZENSHIP STATUS ☐ CITIZEN ☐ |

EXEMPTS: ☐ (DATE THAT EMPLOYEE MUST TERMINATE OR TRANSFER FROM THIS POSITION)

| 24. HRS./WK. | 25. OVERTIME ☐ EXEMPT ☐ NON-EX. |

| 21. DATE STARTED | 22. NATURE OF EMPLOYMENT ☐ NEW HIRE ☐ REINSTATE ☐ REHIRE ☐ SUPPL. POSITION | 23. DURATION OF EMPLOYMENT ☐ PERMANENT ☐ TEMP. AS LOA RELIEF ☐ TEMPORARY IN TAP ☐ TEMP. IN PERM. POS. UNTIL _____ |

| 26. POSITION # | 27. GRADE | 28. STARTING SALARY $ _____ / _____ AT _____ STEP | 29. NEXT SALARY REVIEW FOR $ _____ DATE _____ | 30. BARGAINING UNIT STATUS ☐ MANDATORY ☐ NON-UNION ☐ OPTIONAL |

31. ADDRESS

32. ENTITLEMENTS, SPECIAL BENEFITS, TAX STATUS, ETC,

33. MISCELLANEOUS INFORMATION AND SPECIAL INSTRUCTIONS

ROOM ASST. _____ $ _____

| 34. NEW POSITION ACKNOWLEDGED | DATE | 35. EMPLOYMENT APPROVED | DATE | 36. CLASSIFICATION & SALARY APPROVED | DATE | 37. RECORDED BY PERSONNEL | DATE | 38. RECORDED BY PAYROLL | DATE |

PAYROLL COPY

P-112 (REV. 1-65)
5M 6-68 LAUR.

warding the remaining four to the personnel department. With the appropriate authorizations (approval of the wage and salary administrator and appropriate administrative individuals), the employment section uses this requisition as an authorization to recruit for the position. After an applicant is hired, the bottom of the form is completed with the information identifying the new employee and all necessary information to effect his "put-on." One copy is then forwarded to the payroll department to initiate the put-on; the second copy is filed in the employee's permanent personnel folder; the third copy is returned to the originating department which may at that time destroy the original copy retained when the request was initiated. The final copy is used in the case of an employee who is paid from special funds—moneys received under grants. This copy is forwarded to the fund accounting section.

In advance of the recruitment a *permanent position record* establishing the new position is completed by the records clerk. This is filed in the departmental record drawer and indicates the establishment of a new position in the table of organization for that department. Before filing the personnel copy in the employee's permanent folder, the records clerk completes a permanent employment record card. When an individual is hired, the employment record is placed into the permanent position record after making the appropriate recording on the permanent position record for the individual who has been hired to fill that position.

A permanent folder is completed and made part of the active files for the new employee. All pertinent personnel information is filed in this permanent file during the course of an individual's employment with the institution.

The *personnel action form* (see Exhibit 11, page 99) serves as the document to request changes in status such as reclassification, transfer, salary increase and termination. It, too, is made up in sets of five with distribution similar to that for the personnel requisition form. A manual program such as that described above can use Cardex units to file employee records for ease of finding and filing. Some institutions have devised highly sophisticated computer-based programs for wage and salary administration. Such systems are best developed in conjunction with the payroll system in order to ensure accurate information in both departments. Most successful computerized personnel systems have as their foundation personnel department control over input. Information from the initial establishment of the job to "put-on" of personnel to changes in status are keypunched by operators within the personnel department.

Exhibit 11

THE MOUNT SINAI HOSPITAL
PERSONNEL ACTION FORM

EFFECTIVE DATE	LAST NAME	FIRST NAME	LIFE NO.	DATE HIRED	DATE TYPED

INDICATE ACTION TO BE TAKEN:

☐ TRANSFER
☐ RECLASSIFICATION
☐ CHANGE IN HOURS/SHIFT
☐ TERMINATION

☐ REGULAR MERIT INCREASE
☐ SPECIAL MERIT INCREASE
☐ PROMOTIONAL INCREASE
☐ BARGAINING UNIT INCREASE

☐ OTHER CHANGE IN STATUS __ EXPLAIN
(i.e., LEAVE OF ABSENCE, EXTENSION OF TAP, ETC)

LAST DAY WORKED _____

Change	DEPARTMENT	JOB CLASS. TITLE	HOURS	SHIFT	FUND #	POSITION CODE #	L.G.	SALARY	WEEKLY / BIWEEKLY
FROM								$	☐ WEEKLY ☐ BIWEEKLY
TO								$	☐ WEEKLY ☐ BIWEEKLY

REMARKS OR SPECIAL INSTRUCTIONS:

CANCEL POS #	LIVES IN $	NEXT SALARY REVIEW DATE

LEAVE OF ABSENCE: FROM _____ TO _____

REASON: _____

TERMINATION RECORD

RATING	EXCEL	GOOD	FAIR	POOR
EFFICIENCY	☐	☐	☐	☐
ATTITUDE	☐	☐	☐	☐
ATTENDANCE	☐	☐	☐	☐

RESIGNATION ☐
DISCHARGE ☐
TEMP. EMPL. ☐
OTHER ☐

REASON FOR TERMINATION

☐ REHIRE, IF POSSIBLE   ☐ DO NOT REHIRE

_____ DAYS VACATION DUE   _____ DAYS IN LIEU OF NOTICE

APPROVALS

DEPT. HD./SPVR./PRINC. INVESTIGATOR _____ DATE _____

ASST. DIRECTOR/FUND ACCT. _____

ASSOCIATE DIRECTOR _____

PERSONNEL _____

DIRECTOR _____

RECORDED	
PERSONNEL BY: DATE:	PAYROLL BY: DATE:

PAYROLL COPY

FORM P-111

Personnel Reports

The wage and salary division is responsible for control over the author-ized table of organization. A report of the status of the table of organization, by department, and a comparison of the authorized total for the previous month with the figure for the same month of the previous year should be issued each month. This report provides the count on positions actually filled in each department. It is an invaluable aid to administration. Through a well-staffed and competent records management section of the wage and salary administration division, the table of organization can be carefully controlled. Overlapping positions, positions without proper authorization, employee grievances based upon missed review dates and overpayment or underpayment of employees within a classification are either minimized or prevented.

There is no substitute for a carefully devised wage and salary program which develops up-to-date job descriptions and evaluates positions based upon a recognized job evaluation program. A further appendage of the successful administration of wages and salaries is up-to-date surveys of current market rates. All this can only be accomplished with a complete and modern records system. The wage and salary administrator must present to the administrators facts on the location and classification of jobs, salaries of incumbents and histories of employees. It is not enough merely to develop a program; such a program must be maintained effectively in a current condition.

Conclusion

The cycle which started with job analysis resulting in job descriptions and specifications, which in turn generated a job evaluation program, now comes to its natural conclusion. Remembering that salaries constitute ap-proximately 70 percent of the health care industry's total budget, it becomes necessary for administrators to implement sound controls. Nothing less than an orderly, well-supervised system can be accepted by hospitals' and homes' boards and administrators. The inherent dangers in an informal, poorly administered wage and salary program are the erosion of budgets and the kindling of employee dissatisfaction. Labor costs should be planned and controlled through orderly evaluation and maintenance.

Notes

1. Glenn T. Fischback, "Specific Job Evaluation Systems in Action: American Industrial Man-agement," in Milton L. Rock, *Handbook of Wage and Salary Administration* (New York: McGraw-Hill Book Company, 1972), p. 2-77.

2. E. Lanham, *Job Evaluation* (New York: McGraw-Hill Book Company, 1955), p. 65.

3. Henry A. Sargent, "Using the Point Method to Measure Jobs," in Rock, *op. cit.,* p. 2-33.

4. *Idem.*

5. For an excellent description of the factor comparison method, see Eugene J. Benge, "Using Factor Methods to Measure Jobs," in Rock, *op. cit.,* pp. 2-42 to 2-55.

6. The author wishes to acknowledge the work done by George Kaufman Associates, New York City, in developing the manuals used by The Mount Sinai Hospital.

7. Charles W. Brennan, *Wage Administration* (Homewood, Ill.: Richard D. Irwin, Inc., 1963), p. 3.

8. John A. Patton, C. L. Littlefield, and Stanley Allen Self, *Job Evaluation* (Homewood, Ill.: Richard D. Irwin, Inc., 1964), p. 3.

9. Lawrence C. Lovejoy, *Wage and Salary Administration* (New York: Ronald Press Co., 1959), pp. 294-5.

10. J. Lester Otis and Richard Leukart, *Job Evaluation* (Englewood Cliffs, N.J.: Prentice-Hall, 1954). pp. 420-2.

11. Lovejoy, *op. cit.,* pp. 321-3.

12. Donald R. Thompson, "Solving Problems in Establishing the Pay Structure," in Milton L. Rock, *Handbook of Wage and Salary Administration* (New York: McGraw-Hill Company, 1972), p. 4-21.

13. Glenn A. Bassett and Harvard Y. Weatherbee, *Personnel Systems and Data Management* (New York: American Management Association, 1971), pp. 132-3.

ADDENDA

ADDENDUM A

<u>FACTORS AND DEGREES FOR RATING HOURLY POSITIONS</u>

<u>Introduction</u>. Included in this Section are the definitions of Factors and Degrees to be used in rating all occupations which fall into hourly or non-exempt categories.

<u>Factor 1 - Education or Basic Knowledge</u>. This factor appraises the requirements for the job for the use of shop, trade, technical, or laboratory knowledge, gained through formal education, special courses, or guided apprenticeships or training.

<u>1st Degree</u>: Requires the ability to read, write, and use simple arithmetic.

<u>2nd Degree</u>: Requires the use of arithmetic, the use of simple measuring instruments, together with simple procedural instructions, equivalent to two years of high school.

<u>3rd Degree</u>: Requires the use of fairly complicated instructions, advanced medical technology and arithmetic, use of hand-book formulas, variety of precision measuring or therapeutic instruments, precision diagnostic instruments, complicated office machines such as IBM equipment, trade knowledge in a specialized field or process, equivalent to four years of high school or two years of high school plus two to three years of trade or technical training.

<u>4th Degree</u>: Requires the use of complicated drawings, specifications, advanced mathematics or complicated formulae, a wide variety of precision instruments, broad shop, technical or trade knowledge. Usually equivalent to four years of high school plus four years formal trade, technical or shop training.

<u>5th Degree</u>: Requires a basic technical knowledge sufficient to deal with complicated and involved problems of a semi-professional character or engineering problems. Equivalent to fours years of technical university training.

<u>Factor 2 - Experience</u>. This factor appraises the length of time required by an individual, with the specified education or trade

knowledge to learn to perform the work effectively. Apprenticeships or on-the-job instruction, which have been rated under education, should not be included here. Under Experience include only the time required to attain production standards gained on the job itself or from previous experience on related' or subordinate jobs.

1st Degree: Up to three months.

2nd Degree: Over three months, up to one year.

3rd Degree: Over one year, up to three years.

4th Degree: Over three years, up to five years.

5th Degree: Over five years.

Factor 3 - Initiative and Ingenuity. This factor appraises the independent action, exercise of judgment, making of decisions, or the amount of planning and control which the job requires. Also this factor appraises the degree of complexity of the work.

1st Degree: Requires the ability to understand and follow simple directions, the use of simple equipment involving few decisions and in which the employee is told exactly what to do.

2nd Degree: Requires the ability to work from detailed instructions and the making of minor decisions involving the use of some judgment where the results are subject to immediate check before action is taken.

3rd Degree: Requires the ability to plan and perform a sequence of operations or procedures where standard procedures or recognized methods of operations are available and where it is necessary to make general decisions as to quality, procedure, tolerance limits and set-up sequence.

4th Degree: Requires the ability to plan and perform unusual and difficult work where only general methods of operation, or reference standardized procedures are available and the making of decisions is involved.

5th Degree: Requires outstanding ability to work independently toward general results, where standard procedures and methods of operation are not always available, devise new methods, meeting new conditions, necessitating a high degree of ingenuity, initiative and judgment on very involved and complex tasks.

Factor 4 - Physical Demand. This factor appraises the amount of continuity of physical effort required. Consider the effort expended handling material, machines, and equipment, the weight and frequency of handling, and the periods of unoccupied time.

1st Degree: Light work requiring little physical effort, usually calls for intermittent sitting and standing with only occasional walking throughout the day.

2nd Degree: Light physical effort, working with lightweight materials, or occasionally with average weight materials, use tools or equipment where machine or equipment time exceeds handling time. Some reaching, pushing, lifting, carrying, manipulating, stooping, bending required.

3rd Degree: Sustained physical effort requiring continuity of effort, working with light or average weight material, equipment, animals, etc. Usually short cycle work requiring continuous activity or the operation of several machines or pieces of equipment, or the conduct of several tests where the handling time is equivalent to the total test or machine time, or requiring continuous walking.

4th Degree: Considerable physical effort, working with average or heavy weight material such as patients, animals or or continuous strain of a difficult work position.

5th Degree: Continuous physical exertion working with heavy weight material such as large quantities of food, meat, laundry, furniture, equipment, etc. Work with constant physical strain or intermittent severe strain.

Factor 5 - Mental or Visual Coordination. This factor appraises the degree of mental or visual concentration and coordination required in performing the service or job. Consider the alertness or attention necessary, the length of the task cycle, the coordination of manual dexterity with visual or mental attention.

1st Degree: The service or operation is practically automatic, requiring little mental and only intermittent visual attention.

2nd Degree: Frequent mental or visual attention where the patient service, or the work flow is intermittent, requiring little attention or checking.

3rd Degree: Continuous mental or visual attention where the operation, service, or task is repetitive and requires constant alertness.

4th Degree: Must concentrate mental and visual attention and coordinating closely, both for planning and for accomplishing complex work, or for coordinating a high degree of manual dexterity with close visual attention for sustained period.

5th Degree: Mental or visual attention usually visualizing, planning and conducting highly involved or complex tasks.

Factor 6 - Responsibility for Equipment or Process. This factor appraises responsibility inherent in the job for preventing damage through carelessness to equipment, or time lost from incorrectly performing or following a process for which he is responsible. Amount is that resulting from any one loss, based on probability of occurrence, of equipment or process time only.

1st Degree: Probable damage is negligible.

2nd Degree: Probable damage is seldom more than $25.

3rd Degree: Probable damage is seldom more than $250.

4th Degree: Probable damage is seldom more than $1,000.

5th Degree: Probable damage exceedingly high, reaching several thousand dollars.

Factor 7 - Responsibility for Material. This factor appraises the responsibility for preventing waste or loss through carelessness of materials, such as animals, food, medicinals, etc. Consider the probable number of such items which may be lost, destroyed, spoiled, or damaged before detection and correction in any one situation, the value of the material and time that has gone into its handling, and the possibility of salvage. Avoid use of either maximum or minimum, but try to strike an average based on normal expectation.

1st Degree: Probable loss is seldom over $10.

2nd Degree: Probable loss is seldom over $100.

3rd Degree: Probable loss is seldom more than $250.

4th Degree: Probable loss is seldom more than $500.

5th Degree: Probable loss is very high, up to several thousand dollars.

Factor 8 - Responsibility for the Safety, Comfort, Health or Welfare of Others. This factor appraises the care which must be exercised to prevent injury, discomfort, impairment of health, safety, or welfare of others, and the probable extent of such injury, or impairment. This does not cover injury to employee himself on the job, which is rated under Unavoidable Hazards. Consider possible accidents, etc., to others resulting from error in, or the carelessness in use of equipment, administration of food or medicines, etc. Consider whether other employees, the public, patients, etc., could be injured by carelessness on the job, and, if so, how.

1st Degree: Little responsibility for safety, comfort, etc., of others. Job is performed in an isolated location, or where no equipment, machinery, or patients are involved and the material worked with is very light.

2nd Degree: Only reasonable care to own work is necessary to prevent injury, discomfort, etc., to others or to prevent accidents; if they should arise, accidents would be likely to be minor in nature and not seriously involve the health, safety, or well-being of others.

3rd Degree: Compliance with standard safety and related precautions, in which employee is thoroughly indoctrinated, is necessary to prevent lost-time accidents, disabling or extending discomfort, or health of patients and others.

4th Degree: Constant care is necessary to prevent serious situations arising that might affect patients and others, due to inherent hazards of the job, but where such others may act to prevent their being hurt, disabled, discomforted, etc.

5th Degree: Safety, health, well-being of patients and others depends entirely on correct action of employee on the job being rated, and carelessness may result in fatal accidents, injury, or completely disabling situations.

Factor 9 - Responsibility for the Work of Others. This factor appraises the responsibility which goes with the job for helping, instructing, or assisting the work of others. It is not intended to appraise supervisory responsibility.

1st Degree: Responsibility is solely for one's own work.

2nd Degree: Responsible for instructing, directing, or assisting the work of one or two helpers.

3rd Degree: Responsible for instructing, directing, or assisting the work of a small group of employees and/or helpers in the same occupation, up to ten persons.

4th Degree: Responsible for instructing, directing, and maintaining the flow of work in a group of employees up to 25 persons.

5th Degree: Responsible for instructing, directing, and maintaining the flow of work in a group of more than 25 persons.

Factor 10 - Working Conditions. This factor appraises the surroundings or physical conditions under which the job must be performed and the extent to which those conditions make the job disagreeable. Consider the presence, relative amount of, and continuity of exposure to dust, dirt, heat, fumes, odors, noise, vibration, wet and damp conditions, etc.

1st Degree: Ideal working conditions. Complete absence of any disagreeable elements relating to working conditions.

2nd Degree: Good working conditions. May be slightly dirty or involve occasional exposure to some of the elements listed above. Typical working conditions in a hospital where work does expose employee to a patient-care situation in which he is directly involved.

3rd Degree: Somewhat disagreeable working conditions due to frequent exposure to one or more of the elements listed above, but where these elements are not continuous, if several are present.

4th Degree: Continuous exposure to several disagreeable elements or to one element which is particularly disagreeable.

5th Degree: Continuous and intensive exposure to several extremely disagreeable elements.

Factor 11 - Unavoidable Hazards. This factor appraises the hazards, both to accidental injury or to health, connected with or surrounding the job, even though all health protection rules are followed and all possible safety devices are installed. Consider the material being handled, the possible exposure to deadly or illness-provoking germs, the machines or tools being used, the work position, the possibility of accident, etc., even though none may have, as yet, occurred.

1st Degree: Accident or health hazards negligible.

2nd Degree: Accidents or health hazards improbable, aside from minor injuries, abrasions, cuts, bruises, colds, etc.

3rd Degree: Exposure to lost-time accidents, serious illness, etc., such as crushed hand, foot, loss of fingers, eye injuries from flying particles, exposure to occupational disease, not incapacitating in nature.

4th Degree: Exposure to incapacitating accident or health hazards, as loss of arm or leg, impairment of vision, disabling illness, etc.

5th Degree: Exposure to accidents or occupational disease which may result in total disability or death.

BENCH-MARK JOBS FOR HOURLY POSITION FACTORS AND DEGREES

Factor 1 - Education

1st Degree

MECHANIC (HELPER) E
MAINTENANCE C
LAUNDRY WORKER B
FOOD PREPARER D

2nd Degree

MECHANIC C
PRINTER B
DIETITIAN (HELPER) D
REGISTRAR C

<u>3rd Degree</u>	MECHANIC A NURSE (PRACTICAL) E REGISTRAR B STENOGRAPHER
<u>4th Degree</u>	LABORATORY TECHNICIAN B
<u>5th Degree</u>	LABORATORY TECHNICIAN A

<u>Factor 2 - Experience</u>

<u>1st Degree</u>	MAINTENANCE B LAUNDRY WORKER B DIETITIAN (HELPER) D NURSING AUXILIARY B
<u>2nd Degree</u>	MECHANIC B MAINTENANCE B LAUNDRY WORKER A FOOD PREPARER C
<u>3rd Degree</u>	LABORATORY TECHNICIAN A TELEPHONE OPERATOR B TELEPHONE OPERATOR C
<u>4th Degree</u>	MECHANIC A
<u>5th Degree</u>	

<u>Factor 3 - Initiative and Ingenuity</u>

<u>1st Degree</u>	MECHANIC (HELPER) E MAINTENANCE C FOOD PREPARER D PHARMACIST (HELPER) E
<u>2nd Degree</u>	MECHANIC D LAUNDRY WORKER B DIETITIAN (HELPER) D NURSE (PRACTICAL) E
<u>3rd Degree</u>	MECHANIC A CLERK TYPIST A CUSTODIAN B LABORATORY TECHNICIAN

4th Degree

5th Degree

Factor 4 - Physical Demand

1st Degree   REGISTRAR B

2nd Degree   DIETITIAN (HELPER) D
PHARMACIST (HELPER) E
LABORATORY TECHNICIAN A
STENOGRAPHER

3rd Degree   MECHANIC A
MAINTENANCE B
LAUNDRY WORKER A
FOOD PREPARER C

4th Degree   MECHANIC D
MAINTENANCE C

5th Degree

Factor 5 - Mental or Visual Coordination

1st Degree   REGISTRAR C

2nd Degree   MECHANIC (HELPER) E
DIETITIAN (HELPER) D
NURSING AUXILIARY B

3rd Degree   MECHANIC A
MAINTENANCE A
LAUNDRY WORKER A
FOOD PREPARER C

4th Degree

5th Degree

ADDENDUM A *(Cont'd)*

Factor 6 - Responsibility for Equipment	
<u>1st Degree</u>	MECHANIC (HELPER) E DIETITIAN (HELPER) D NURSE (PRACTICAL) E REGISTRAR C
<u>2nd Degree</u>	MECHANIC C MAINTENANCE C LAUNDRY WORKER A FOOD PREPARER C
<u>3rd Degree</u>	MECHANIC B PROJECTIONIST
<u>4th Degree</u>	
<u>5th Degree</u>	MECHANIC A
Factor 7 - Responsibility for Materials	
<u>1st Degree</u>	MECHANIC A MAINTENANCE B LAUNDRY WORKER B DIETITIAN (HELPER) D
<u>2nd Degree</u>	FOOD PREPARER C LABORATORY TECHNICIAN A STOREROOM ATTENDANT A
<u>3rd Degree</u>	LAUNDRY WORKER A
<u>4th Degree</u>	
<u>5th Degree</u>	
Factor 8 - Responsibility for Safety of Others	
<u>1st Degree</u>	FOOD PREPARER D CLERK TYPIST A TELEPHONE OPERATOR B PRINTER B
<u>2nd Degree</u>	MECHANIC C LAUNDRY WORKER A DIETITIAN (HELPER) D NURSING AUXILIARY C

3rd Degree	MECHANIC A
	MAINTENANCE B
	AUXILIARY NURSE A
	LABORATORY TECHNICIAN B
4th Degree	NURSE (PRACTICAL) E
	CUSTODIAN B
5th Degree	

Factor 9 - Responsibility for Work of Others

1st Degree	MECHANIC (HELPER) E
	MAINTENANCE C
	LAUNDRY WORKER C
	FOOD PREPARER D
2nd Degree	MECHANIC A
	LAUNDRY WORKER A
	DIETITIAN (HELPER) D
	NURSE (PRACTICAL) E
3rd Degree	MAINTENANCE A
	TELEPHONE OPERATOR B
	STOREROOM ATTENDANT A
4th Degree	
5th Degree	

Factor 10 - Working Conditions

1st Degree	CLERK TYPIST A
	CLERK
2nd Degree	MAINTENANCE B
	DIETITIAN (HELPER) D
	NURSE (PRACTICAL) E
	PHARMACIST (HELPER) E
3rd Degree	MECHANIC A
	LAUNDRY WORKER A
	FOOD PREPARER C
	LABORATORY TECHNICIAN (HELPER) D

4th Degree

5th Degree

Factor 11 - Unavoidable Hazards

1st Degree   REGISTRAR B
STENOGRAPHER
TELEPHONE OPERATOR B
CLERK TYPIST A

2nd Degree   MECHANIC (HELPER) E
MAINTENANCE B
DIETITIAN (HELPER) D
NURSE (PRACTICAL) E

3rd Degree   MECHANIC A
LAUNDRY WORKER A
LABORATORY TECHNICIAN (HELPER) D
NURSING AUXILIARY A

4th Degree

5th Degree

Key to Grades for Hourly Positions

Grade	Point Range
11	151 and under
10	152-173
9	174-195
8	196-217
7	218-239
6	240-261
5	262-283
4	284-305
3	306-327
2	328-349
1	350-371

ADDENDUM B

ESTABLISHMENT OF NEW POSITIONS * Page 1	Issued: Revised:

The following procedure describes the st′ps that must be taken to
add a new position to a department's table of organization.

4.51 A department head may request a new position in the following
situations:

    4.511 Work volume has materially and permanently increased due
to additional functions assumed by the department. Under
these circumstances a request may be made for a "newly
authorized position" (NAP).

    4.512 Work volume has temporarily or seasonally increased
or the department has undertaken a special project
or temporarily assumed additional functions. Under
these circumstances a request may be made for a
"temporarily authorized position" (TAP). A TAP
may be authorized up to a maximum of one year.

    4.513 An additional employee is required for coverage during
a vacation period. In this case a request may be made
for a "vacation relief position" (VRP).

    4.514 A request for "LOA relief" coverage is not handled as a
request for a new position. An employee hired to fill
a position whose incumbent is on leave of absence is
assigned to that same position. LOA relief requisitions
should therefore be handled according to Personnel Policy
#4.6, "Employment Action for Existing Positions."

    4.515 Where the situation requires less than a full-time addition
to the department's T.O., the request may be for a
"part-time NAP," "part-time TAP," or "part-time VRP"
as appropriate.

4.52 A request for a new position should be initiated by the use of a
"Personnel Requisition," Form No. P-112. (A sample of this
form is appended.) Supplies are available from the Storeroom.

4.53 The following steps are necessary to obtain authorization for a
new position:

    4.531 Complete sections 1, 2, 3 - Date, Signature, Department.

* Excerpt

ADDENDUM C

		Issued:
COMPENSATION STANDARDS* Page 1		Revised:

The following policy statements outline the standards and requirements for wage and salary compensation at the Institution.

7.11 The Institution will maintain salaries competitive with those prevailing for comparable jobs in health care institutions in the Greater New York area.

7.12 An equitable compensation structure will be maintained for the Institution's numerous jobs based on relative responsibility, knowledge and skill requirements, working conditions and other job characteristics.

7.13 Employees not covered by collective bargaining agreements requiring fixed wages and increments will be given increases based on individual performance.

7.14 Bargaining unit employees will receive wages and increments as required by contract.

7.15 Mount Sinai will comply with all legal requirements affecting employee compensation.

7.16 A formal wage and salary administration program is to be maintained including such elements as:

    7.161 Job Descriptions setting forth job content, qualification requirements, job classification and salary grade;

    7.162 Job Analysis providing systematic study of jobs by cross-comparison of compensable job factors;

    7.163 Salary Survey to ascertain prevailing salaries paid by other employers for comparable jobs;

    7.164 Job Evaluation to determine the relative compensability of individual positions;

    7.165 Job Classification to categorize groups of related positions;

    7.166 Salary Grading to assign specific salary rates and ranges to job classifications;

*Excerpt

ADDENDUM D

MERIT INCREASES *	Issued:
Page 1	Revised:

The following statements describe the Institution's policy and procedure regarding salary increases based on employee performance.

7.31 Periodic increases for bargaining unit employees are determined by collective bargaining agreement. Because such agreements ordinarily require automatic increases irrespective of individual performance, merit increases are not provided for bargaining unit employees in addition to the contractual increases.

7.32 Merit increases for non-bargaining unit employees are ordinarily given each July. Within each salary grade, merit increases may be in variable amounts depending on the employee's job performance.

    7.321 The amount of increase for a non-bargaining unit employee hired less than a year before the increase date may be adjusted in accordance with the number of months of employment. Employees who have served less than 3 months before their first July increase date ordinarily will not receive an increase.

7.33 Periodic and merit increases for all employees of a department are subject to approved departmental budgetary allocations. Significant deviations must be discussed with cognizant administrative staff members.

7.34 Every June, the Wage and Salary Section will send each department a list of bargaining unit and non-bargaining unit employees. The bargaining unit list will indicate the current and the new salary rates. The non-bargaining unit list will indicate the current rates with provision for the department to indicate the new rates (except for professional nursing staff, house staff, and social workers whose increases are fixed).

7.35 Special merit increases, i.e., extraordinary performance increases requested, other than on the July 1st review date, or in greater than the maximum amount for the salary grade, must be approved by all cognizant administrative staff including the Director of the Hospital or the Dean of the School of Medicine, or their designeees, as appropriate.

7.36 Red-circle increases, i.e., increases bringing an employee's salary above the maximum of his range, require the same level of approval as in #7.35.

*Excerpt

119

IV. RECRUITMENT, SCREENING AND SELECTION

Personnel Managers and other department heads must utilize every possible technique to locate, screen and select people they need. If they are going to be successful, they must reexamine their personnel practices. If jobs are not filled, if new and dynamic people are not attracted to a company, the policies muet be changed. A company cannot survive without the human resources to keep it alive, vigorous and growing.[1]

Effective recruiting involves a determination of future needs, the clear definition and description of the types of people needed and an evaluation and determination of methods to be used in each particular case. In addition, it includes an investigation of the whole process of demand and supply. The most marked of changes in employment methods over the years has been the establishment of centralized screening and decentralized hiring. When the personnel department receives a requisition, several questions must be answered immediately: What are the specific job requirements for this position? What kind of person must be found to meet these requirements? Where should the department start looking to find an individual who matches these requirements?

Recruitment

Recruitment is a positive mechanism. It involves finding applicants and encouraging potential employees to seek jobs at a specific institution. Before establishing a sound recruitment program, it is important that the sources of personnel are identified. Some of these sources are:

1. Present employees.
2. Employee referrals.
3. Applicants at the gate.
4. Write-ins.
5. Public employment agencies.
6. Private employment agencies.
7. Unions.
8. Retired military personnel.
9. Other retired individuals.
10. Schools and colleges.

121

Present Employees

Most institutions agree that promotions from within encourage present staff members to be more efficient and, indeed, kindle the spark of motivation present in all employees. The institution is offered a candidate for the position whose record is well-known. By using the mechanisms of transfer and promotion, lower-level jobs become available which the institution may find easier to fill. Careful consideration should be given to the procedure for effecting the fullest possible use of internal sources. This procedure would include:

1. Job posting.
2. Use of personnel records.
3. Skill banks.
4. Reemployment of former employees.

Job posting developed in many institutions through union pressures. It can be as effective in a nonunionized institution as in a unionized one. It is a practice found in many successful enterprises where preference is given to present employees in all opportunities for transfers and promotions. The usual procedure is to post the job on bulletin boards throughout the institution and include a brief description of the requirements. A concomitant instrument in effecting a successful job posting program is a specific personnel policy covering the criteria for promotion and transfers (see Exhibit 1, pages 124-125). In addition, an application for transfer (see Exhibit 2, page 126) is a useful form and should include the supervisor's recommendation regarding the employee's qualifications. The employee's personnel record files can be very effective in determining the past record of an applicant for transfer and promotion. The employee's prior experience can be ascertained by a review of these records. Skill banks have been developed by many institutions to obviate unnecessary recruitment on the outside for skills that are available internally. Information on previous skills of present employees may be developed into computerized rosters from which lists of employees who have a specific skill can be made available at times of recruitment for specific job opportunities. The reemployment of former employees is facilitated by keeping up-to-date lists of employees who have been either laid off or voluntarily terminated. Several institutions have successfully recruited registered nurses by reviewing past records of terminations in the nursing department and communicating with each qualified nurse who voluntarily terminated over the past five years.

It is well to keep in mind the reluctance of supervisors to facilitate transfers or promotions of employees from a job in their department to a higher-rated job in another department. A good employee, both well-motivated and efficient, is a precious commodity which some supervisors feel must be protected and hoarded at all costs. It is important that the institution educate its supervisors to prevent blocking of transfers and promotions for qualified employees. A supervisor who permits and encourages upward mobility will build a well-motivated and efficient work force.

Employee Referrals

Experience has indicated that present employees are an excellent source for referral of qualified applicants for openings in their own institution. It is not surprising that present employees will carefully pre-screen any applicant whom they refer for employment to their institution. They seldom are willing to engender the criticism and embarrassment that may develop from referring an unqualified applicant. There is little question that morale is boosted when employees find that their recommendations are considered and accepted. It also follows that if an employee is dissatisfied with his job, he will not refer his friends or relatives for employment. Again, positions are posted in such a program and announcements of openings are made through the various employee communication vehicles. Some of the more successful nurse recruitment programs have incorporated bonuses for employees who refer nurses for employment. One institution offered $100 for each registered nurse referred by an employee and hired. This method of hiring is relatively inexpensive and can add to the overall good will in the institution. It is important that rejections of candidates referred by present employees are handled in the most careful and considerate manner. Reasons for the rejection should be clearly communicated to both the candidate and his sponsor.

Applicants at the Gate

Probably the largest single source of candidates is those who apply to the institution's employment office without any formal solicitation on the part of the institution. They do not involve any recruitment cost for the institution and often are attracted to applying for positions by the reputation of that institution. Since they are not responding to a specific solicitation, the institution is often faced with applicants for nonexisting positions. It behooves the employer to arrange for brief interviews even if positions are not available in order to generate good will within the community. This is an investment for future recruitment needs.

Exhibit 1

PERSONNEL POLICY # 6.1	
PROMOTIONS AND TRANSFERS - CRITERIA* Page 1	Issued: 11/1/70 Revised:

The following statements describe the bases upon which employee promotions and transfers are made.

6.11 Definition of Promotion: Promotion is defined as the permanent
reassignment of an employee to work at a higher job classification
and compensation rate. Promotion occurs when:

6.111 the employee transfers to a higher position (promotional
transfer);

6.112 the employee's present position is reclassified upward.

(See also Personnel Policy #7.4, "Promotional Increases,"
and Personnel Policy #7.6, "Reclassification").

6.12 Definition of Transfer: Transfer is defined as the permanent
movement of an employee from one position to another. If the
move is to a higher position, it is considered a promotional
transfer. Transfers are further distinguished as:

6.121 intradepartmental, i.e., where the transfer is within the
department;

6.122 interdepartmental, i.e., where the transfer is to a different department.

6.13 Criteria for Promotion: Where a promotional vacancy occurs
and two or more employees are under consideration, the
following factors are considered in selection:

6.131 For bargaining unit positions, the employee with the
greatest classification seniority will be promoted,
unless there is an appreciable difference in their
ability to do the work. If there is such a difference,
the more able employee will be promoted.

6.132 For non-bargaining unit positions, ability to do the
work and classification seniority are considered.
Where ability is relatively equal, the senior employee
is promoted. The Medical Center is the sole judge of

MOUNT SINAI MEDICAL CENTER

*Excerpt

Exhibit 1 *(Cont'd)*

PERSONNEL POLICY # 6.2	
PROMOTIONS AND TRANSFERS - PROCEDURE Page 1	Issued: 11/1/70 Revised:

The following statements describe the steps to be taken and requirements to be observed in selecting employees for promotions and transfers. (In this Policy Statement the term "transfer" includes "promotional" as well as "lateral" transfers. It does not include shift changes.)

6.21 <u>Notification of Vacant Positions</u>: The Employment Section maintains a register of vacant positions. Where appropriate, vacancies are posted on Medical Center bulletin boards. Information on non-posted vacancies is available from the Employment Section.

6.22 <u>Discussion Between Employee and Supervisor</u>: An employee who wishes to apply for promotion or transfer to another position should discuss his intentions with his supervisor before making formal application.

6.23 <u>Discussion Between Supervisors</u>: A supervisor who wishes to consider an employee for promotion or transfer from another department should discuss his intentions with the candidate's supervisor and with the Employment Manager before he makes an overture to the candidate.

6.24 <u>Application Procedure</u>: If the employee's experience and performance suggests that he might be a suitable candidate for the position he seeks, the employee and his supervisor should jointly prepare an Application for Transfer (form P-140, sample appended, available from the Employment Office) and forward this form to the Employment Manager.

    6.241 The supervisor should complete the identifying information on Part I of the form. The employee should specify the "nature of transfer requested" and "reason for transfer request." The employee should enter his signature and date.

    6.242 The supervisor should complete Part II of the form, giving his candid impression of the employee's suitability for the position applied for. He should also indicate the earliest date that the employee may be released from his present position. The supervisor should sign and date the form and send it to the Employment Manager immediately.

Exhibit 2

THE MOUNT SINAI HOSPITAL
NEW YORK

Today's date _____

I APPLICATION FOR TRANSFER: _____
(to be completed by employee and/or superv'r)   Employee's name   Employee #   Date employed

_____   _____   _____   _____
present position   department   supervisor   supervisor's ext.

_____ $ _____ per _____
present shift /hours   present gross salary

1. Nature of transfer requested: ☐ Different type of work (specify) _____

                                         ☐ Different hours (specify) _____

                                         ☐ Different area (specify) _____

                                         ☐ Other (specify) _____

2. Reason for transfer request: ☐ Interest in, and qualifications for other type of work

                                         ☐ Dissatisfaction with present job (explain) _____

                                         ☐ Other (explain) _____

3. Employee's signature _____   Date left with supervisor _____

II SUPERVISOR'S RECOMMENDATIONS: [Candid responses will help the Hospital place and retain qualified employees in appropriate jobs. Every effort should be made to encourage the advancement of competent employees.]

1. If this employee were applying for a transfer to your department, would you accept him? _____
2. Why? _____
3. What is your evaluation of this employee's strengths, and weaknesses, particularly as they may affect the job the employee is applying for? _____

_____

_____

4. If a transfer opportunity materializes, what is the earliest date the employee may be released from his present position?

_____

5. Other remarks: _____

_____

_____

6. Supervisor's signature: _____

Date sent to Employment Section _____

P-140

Write-Ins

A group of applicants similar to those who walk in without solicitation are those who write in without solicitation. Again, prompt and courteous responses to such inquiries are in order. It can be productive to keep a file of such applicants who either walk in or write in and find no positions available. Many employment offices of health care institutions keep up-to-date records of such inquiries. These files are pruned on a regular basis and reviewed when positions do become available.

Public Employment Agencies

A wise man once said you do something well and have several sidelines. The same advice might be given to institutions in meeting their recruitment needs. All possible sources should be explored. Since 1933, larger communities throughout the nation have been served by public employment offices that have been valuable sources of applicants for open positions. These public offices have also been charged with the job of administering unemployment compensation benefits. As a result, they have an added interest in discovering job opportunities for those who are out of work. Employment agencies are a key source of applicants. An institution can place an opening with such an agency, either by telephone or in person. Many of these agencies are equipped to do testing that is invaluable to the smaller health services institutions unable to do such testing on their own. Recently the United States Employment Service introduced a new computerized job bank system. This has increased their effectiveness. Of course, *there is no fee charged to either employers or employees for such services.*

Private Employment Agencies

There are approximately 10,000 private employment agencies in the United States. More and more private employment offices specialize in skilled manual and white-collar manpower. These agencies are an excellent source for the recruitment of personnel for higher level positions. Some of the more sophisticated agencies are using data processing techniques which facilitate the matching of employer requirements and applicants in the file. Many institutions develop close relationships with the private agencies based upon their past success in filling jobs for them. *Where the skills sought are in short supply, the employer usually takes the responsibility for the fee.* In the cases of low-level positions and those skills normally in sufficient supply in the labor market, the applicant pays the fee soon after starting on the job. Some agencies are parts of national chains and, therefore, can call upon branch offices in other cities in searching for applicants. This offers a marked advantage in recruitment of highly specialized categories. In selecting an agency, an institution can be guided by the agency's membership in a state or national association that subscribes to certain professional or ethical standards. A directory of private employment agencies in the United States is published by the National Employment Office, Washington, D. C. 20006. Pell lists certain recommendations in dealing with private employment agencies.[2]

1. DO:
Learn which employment agencies are best for different types of jobs.
Get to know the staff of the agencies with which a company works.
Learn what special or added services agencies offer.
Communicate with the agency—let them have full job specifications and give them feedback on the results of interviews.
Periodically evaluate the success of the agencies with which you work.
Understand the agencies' fee schedule.

2. DO NOT:
List the same job with too many agencies in the same area.
Accept referrals from agencies on applicants previously referred by other sources.
Refer an applicant sent by an agency in whom there is no interest to another employer.
Accept referrals from an agency without a clear understanding regarding who is to pay the fee and how much it will be.

Unions

Institutions having collective bargaining agreements with unions often have available to them union hiring halls. Some contracts provide for such services as the first contact to be made by the employer before hiring from the outside. Clear language should be provided on the options of the employer in using a union hiring hall. The following is a provision of a collective bargaining agreement for the use of a union hiring hall.

1. The institution shall notify the union employment service of all bargaining unit jobs and training position vacancies and shall afford the service 24 hours from the time of notification to refer an applicant for the vacancy before the institution hires from any other source.

2. Neither the union employment service in referring nor the institution hiring shall discriminate against an applicant because of membership or nonmembership in the union.

3. The cost of operating the employment service shall be borne by the union.

4. The institution retains the right to hire such applicants referred by the employment service as it deems qualified in its sole discretion.

5. The institution retains the right to hire applicants from other sources in the event the employment service does not refer qualified applicants within such 24-hour period.

6. The institution shall not be required to notify the employment service of any job vacancy which must be filled without delay in order to meet an emergency or to safeguard the health, safety or well-being of patients.

Retired Military Personnel

Retired military personnel offer a potentially excellent recruitment source, as do veterans released from military service. Many of these individuals are highly qualified and possess skills often not found in the civilian population. The military has expended enormous funds in training such individuals and many of these skills are transferable to civilian occupations. Institutions recruiting such personnel do so by advertisements in military publications and referring job openings to separation centers. The Retired Officers Association in Washington, D.C., is a useful agency to contact. *This agency does not charge any fee.*

Other Retired Individuals

More and more institutions have found a pool of qualified, well-motivated individuals made available by early retirement programs in industry and other institutions. Some of these individuals, often in their early fifties, have retired from positions held for 20 and 30 years and now seek to gain employment in new positions. They offer the institution upwards of ten years of productive working time. There are many Forty-Plus clubs in existence in large cities throughout the country who can provide applicants well-qualified for positions which institutions may have available. *There is no charge for such services.* In addition, handicapped workers offer still another source of productive, well-motivated applicants.

Schools and Colleges

Visits to campuses and high schools have produced excellent candidates for positions in the health service industry. Many institutions have developed programs which provide periodic visits to local schools and colleges at which time general information is provided the senior classes as to opportunities available in the institution. Working closely with the school's placement office, a year-round educational program is possible which can attract highly qualified young applicants. These individuals offer a firm educational base for institutional training programs. In developing a program to recruit graduates of local schools and colleges, it is essential that visits be planned in advance; announcements clearly made to the schools well before the visit; arrangements made for interviewing time and space; and contacts carefully developed with members of the academic community.

Recruitment Advertisement

The most widely used recruitment technique is that of placing classified ads. Two major considerations go into the decision to place a help-wanted ad: (1) the media to be used, and (2) the layout or construction of the ad. The media available to the employer include daily newspapers, weekend newspapers, trade publications and specialized newspapers and magazines. A careful analysis must be undertaken as to the audience reached by each of these media. *As with all other recruitment techniques, it is essential to maintain records which will indicate the success of each of the media based upon the type of skill sought.* Many institutions find trade magazines quite effective for the placement of recruitment advertisements for professional and managerial positions. On the other hand, the help-wanted section of the local newspaper produces best results for nonskilled, low-level applicants.

In deciding upon the construction of the ad, cost and potential results must be carefully weighed. Classified ads are used most frequently because of the low cost involved, while display ads, which are larger and more costly, are used for difficult-to-recruit positions. In some cases blind ads are preferred. These are classified or display ads which do not identify the institution. The applicants are directed to a box number which affords the institution the opportunity to review resumes without the need to communicate rejections to those obviously not qualified. When an institution enjoys a good reputation in the community, the blind ad is not as effective as placement of an ad which identifies the institution. Many qualified applicants are drawn to specific institutions solely on their reputation. Yet there are times when blind ads are essential to preserve the confidential nature of the recruitment since the institution may not want to indicate to present employees or to prospective employees its identity. Some ads ask for reply by letter while others direct the applicant to a phone number. Still others list interviewing hours at specific times for those who wish to respond to an ad. In the construction of an attractive ad that will improve the quality of responses, Pell suggests a system he calls AIDA:[3]

1. *Attention*—one must attract attention to the ad. It must be seen to be

read. Typeface can attract readers. The headline should be one or two words which have pulling power.

2. *Interest*—once the eye has been attracted to the ad, it is essential to develop interest in the job. Salary and fringe benefits are certainly interest factors. Others are special advantages offered, information about the company and opportunities for the geographic area.

3. *Desire*—amplification of the interest factors plus the extras which the job offers in terms of growth, job satisfaction and personal value help create this desire. Readers are more interested in themselves than anything else. Write the ad to appeal to them, not to satisfy the writer's ego.

4. *Action*—not only must the ad be appealing, but also it should instigate action. Give him the name, the phone number and the time the applicant should call.

In addition to advertising of open positions, many institutions have available special recruitment literature for applicants. This literature is usually distributed at the time of the interview but can be forwarded to an applicant in advance of the interview. It should be graphically appealing and contain pertinent information to attract the qualified applicant to the institution.

Selection

While recruitment is a positive mechanism designed to bring in as many applicants as possible, selection can be considered a negative mechanism. A proper selection program lets only the qualified applicants through the sieve. An attempt is made to appraise qualities the institution feels are indicative of success on the job. This process necessitates the making of a value judgment, a forecast as to which applicants will turn out to be productive employees. As with any forecasting there are tools of the trade:

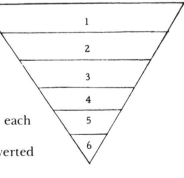

1. The application blank.
2. The interview.
3. Tests.
4. The reference check.
5. The preemployment physical.

The selection process is made up of various stages which should be designed to permit candidates through each phase at a numerically decreasing rate. Calhoun likens the procedure to an inverted triangle:[4]

Application Forms

The application form plays a simple, yet important role in selection. Its contents can discourage unsuitable applicants and its design can reflect the company's dignity, reduce to a minimum the time needed to fill it out and simplify its review. Its wording and its comprehensiveness affect the efficiency and validity of the selection process.[5]

The application blank must be designed for the specific task it is to perform, namely, to improve the selection of applicants. It can, if properly designed, greatly reduce the time required for the interview which will follow its completion. It should provide definitive indicators which an experienced interviewer can quickly interpret. In the final analysis, its primary objective is that of comparing the applicant's qualifications with the qualifications required for the available job. It is the most widely used personnel selection device. Most application blanks contain the following items:

    1. Identifying information:

      a. Name, address, telephone number.

      b. Date of birth, marital status and number of dependents.

      c. Social Security number.

      d. Height, weight and physical characteristics.

    2. Education and training:

      a. Record of grade school, high school, technical or trade school, college and graduate school completion.

      b. Special skills developed through other training.

    3. Work experience:

      a. Prior positions with dates of employment, salary, duties and reason for leaving.

    4. Personal references.

    5. Record of service in the armed forces.

    6. Hobbies and leisure time interests.

In the construction of an application blank, it is important for the institution to carefully review the appropriate state and federal laws affecting questions in application blanks and employment interviews. Exhibit 3 (see pages 148-151) is an example of an all-inclusive application blank.

Three common purposes of the application blank are:[6]

    1. Preliminary screening to determine whether or not an interview is needed.

    2. An interview aid to provide an outline of basic facts which may be elaborated during the interview.

    3. A selection device based on the blank's own merits.

Recent studies indicate that most applicants are relatively honest in reporting work history on application blanks. Although some applicants give advantageously inaccurate replies to reasons for separation, job duties and wages, apparently the implied verification of application facts (which should be clearly stated on the form itself) is a sufficient deterrent to falsification of information. Mandell suggests that the specific application blank which will produce the best results must be designed in relation to the selection methods used and selection ratios which will apply. He states, for example:

1. A brief form will do if the next step in the selection process is an inexpensive written test which will eliminate a large percentage of the applicants.

2. If a resume is requested first, the scope of its contents should be suggested.

3. A biographical information blank reduces the need for depth in the application form.

4. A general application blank can be supplemented by a check list prepared for each type of work to ensure that the applicant has the necessary qualifications.[7]

In constructing an application blank, the designer should not fail to recognize that some applicants will find varying degrees of difficulty and discomfort in their attempt to complete it. It may be necessary to tailor application blanks to the varying levels of applicants that apply to an institution—for example, one for professional employees, a second for semiskilled employees and a third for nonskilled employees. Another consideration is the eventual use of the application blank. Some institutions use the blank as a permanent personnel record; therefore, it must include many items otherwise superfluous for selection and placement. Some application blanks are printed on expensive and thick stock which when folded can be inserted into a Cardex file and may be used for wage and salary administration purposes. Usually where such a decision is made, i.e., *to use it as a permanent personnel record application blank,* the cost of such forms for all applicants becomes prohibitive when one considers a normal selection ratio of 10 applicants for one hire. Therefore, if the institution has made a decision to use a permanent personnel record application blank, it may find a *preliminary short-form application* useful. The preliminary short-form application will elicit key information necessary to make an initial screening to determine if the applicant appears to possess the requisite background for the position available. Then, and only then, the permanent application blank may be completed. Although this practice is not uncommon, it is not the most satisfactory procedure. The permanent personnel record should be separated

Exhibit 3

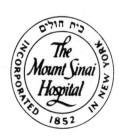

THE MOUNT SINAI MEDICAL CENTER

ONE GUSTAVE L. LEVY PLACE - NEW YORK, N.Y. 10029

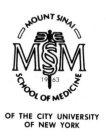

OF THE CITY UNIVERSITY
OF NEW YORK

APPLICATION for EMPLOYMENT

RETURN TO: (check one)

☐ MOUNT SINAI SCHOOL OF MEDICINE EMPLOYMENT OFFICE

☐ MOUNT SINAI HOSPITAL EMPLOYMENT OFFICE

☐ MOUNT SINAI HOSPITAL PROFESSIONAL NURSE
    RECRUITMENT EMPLOYMENT OFFICE

☐ MOUNT SINAI SERVICES EMPLOYMENT OFFICE

EQUAL EMPLOYMENT OPPORTUNITY THROUGH AFFIRMATIVE ACTION

P123 15M 12/77 S.R.C.

Exhibit 3 *(Cont'd)*

THE MOUNT SINAI HOSPITAL AND THE MOUNT SINAI SCHOOL OF MEDICINE OF THE CITY UNIVERSITY OF NEW YORK ARE EQUAL EMPLOYMENT AFFIRMATIVE ACTION EMPLOYERS. PERSONNEL ARE CHOSEN ON THE BASIS OF ABILITY AND QUALIFICATIONS WITHOUT REGARD TO RACE, COLOR, RELIGION, SEX, AGE, NATIONAL ORIGIN, MARITAL STATUS, HANDICAP OR VETERAN STATUS IN COMPLIANCE WITH FEDERAL, STATE, AND MUNICIPAL LAWS.

| NAME (PRINT)   LAST | FIRST | MIDDLE | DATE | SOC. SEC. NO. | POSITION APPLIED FOR |

| ADDRESS | CITY | STATE | ZIP CODE | TEL. NO. | ARE YOU 18 YEARS OR OLDER ☐ YES ☐ NO IF NOT - PLEASE SPECIFY AGE |

CITIZEN OF U.S. ☐ YES ☐ YES ☐ NO IF NOT - DO YOU HAVE LEGAL RIGHT TO WORK IN U.S. ☐ NO
HAVE YOU EVER BEEN EMPLOYED BY MOUNT SINAI- IF YES, INDICATE DATE AND POSITION ☐ YES ☐ NO

DO YOU HAVE ANY RELATIVES EMPLOYED BY MOUNT SINAI OTHER THAN SPOUSE. ☐ NO ☐ YES IF YES - LIST NAMES

YOU MAY NOT BE ASSIGNED TO A POSITION WHERE YOU WOULD SUPERVISE OR BE SUPERVISED BY A RELATIVE.

HOW DID YOU LEARN OF MOUNT SINAI ☐ ADVERTISEMENT ☐ OTHER

TYPE OF POSITION ☐ FULL TIME ☐ PART TIME ☐ TEMPORARY ☐ PERMANENT ☐ SUMMER
SHIFTS AVAIL.   HOURS AVAIL.   DAYS AVAIL.   I AGREE TO ROTATE ALL THREE SHIFTS AS REQUIRED
SIGNATURE

DATE OF U.S. MILITARY SERVICE BRANCH OF U.S. MILITARY SERVICE
WHICH FOREIGN LANGUAGES DO YOU READ AND/OR WRITE AND/OR SPEAK FLUENTLY

SKILLS:
TYPING (SPECIFY) ☐ ELECTRIC ☐ MANUAL ☐ OTHER   W.P.M.
☐ STENO   W.P.M. ☐ DICTAPHONE ☐ MEDICAL TERMINOLOGY
PLEASE LIST OTHER SPECIAL SKILLS

HAVE YOU EVER BEEN CONVICTED OF A CRIME OR OFFENSE OTHER THAN A MINOR TRAFFIC VIOLATION ☐ YES ☐ NO IF YES, PLEASE EXPLAIN:

WHEN   WHERE   DISPOSITION OF OFFENSE

ARE THERE ANY ARRESTS OR CRIMINAL PROCEEDINGS CURRENTLY PENDING AGAINST YOU ☐ NO ☐ YES - IF YES, PLEASE EXPLAIN -

NEW YORK STATE LAW AGAINST DISCRIMINATION PROHIBITS UNJUSTIFIED DISCRIMINATION ON THE BASIS OF A CRIMINAL CONVICTION RECORD

DO YOU HAVE ANY IMPAIRMENTS, PHYSICAL OR MENTAL, WHICH WILL INTERFERE WITH YOUR ABILITY TO PERFORM THE JOB FOR WHICH YOU ARE APPLYING? PLEASE DESCRIBE.

ARE THERE ANY POSITIONS OR TYPES OF POSITIONS FOR WHICH YOU SHOULD NOT BE CONSIDERED OR JOB DUTIES YOU CANNOT PERFORM BECAUSE OF A PHYSICAL OR MENTAL OR MEDICAL DISABILITY. - PLEASE DESCRIBE

EDUCATION	NAME OF SCHOOL	ADDRESS	YEARS COMPLETED	DATE LEFT	IF GRAD. DEG./MAJ.	NOT GRAD. - LEVEL COMPLETED NO. of CREDITS
HIGH SCHOOL or highest grade attended						
COLLEGE/ UNIVERSITY						
TECHNICAL or NURSING SCHOOL						
GRADUATE SCHOOL						

PLEASE LIST PROFESSIONAL LICENSES AND/OR CERTIFICATION BELOW:

TYPE	STATE	EXPIRATION DATE	REGISTRATION NUMBER

Exhibit 3 *(Cont'd)*

THE FOLLOWING SECTION TO BE COMPLETED BY PROFESSIONAL NURSING APPLICANTS ONLY:				
SPECIFY BELOW YOUR PREFERRED AREAS OF CLINICAL NURSING			DESIRE HOUSING	I AGREE TO ROTATE ALL THREE SHIFTS
1.	2.	3.	☐ ☐ YES NO	SIGNATURE

R.N. AND L.P.N.

IF YOU DO NOT HAVE A CURRENT AND VALID N.Y. STATE NURSING LICENSE, HAVE YOU MADE APPLICATION   ☐ NO ☐ YES   WHEN

TYPE - R.N. L.P.N. OTHER............	STATE ISSUED	EXPIRATION DATE	REGISTRATION NO.
1			
2			
3			

EMPLOYMENT HISTORY   PLEASE COMPLETE SECTION EVEN IF YOU ATTACHED RESUME. LIST CURRENT OR MOST RECENT POSITION FIRST AND COVER PERIODS OF EMPLOYMENT FOR THE LAST SEVEN (7) YEARS

FROM / TO	EMPLOYER'S NAME/ADDRESS TEL. NO./SUPERVISOR	POSITION TITLE / JOB DUTIES	REASONS FOR LEAVING
			FINAL SALARY
FROM / TO			REASONS FOR LEAVING
			FINAL SALARY
FROM / TO			REASONS FOR LEAVING
			FINAL SALARY

IS ANY ADDITIONAL INFORMATION RELATIVE TO CHANGE IN NAME, USE OF AN ASSUMED NAME OR NICKNAME NECESSARY TO ENABLE A CHECK ON YOUR WORK RECORD? -IF YES- PLEASE EXPLAIN

DO YOU AUTHORIZE US TO CONTACT YOUR PRESENT EMPLOYER FOR REFERENCE PRIOR TO MOUNT SINAI

EMPLOYMENT   ☐ YES   ☐ NO

AUTHORIZED SIGNATURE

IF EMPLOYER IS NO LONGER IN BUSINESS HOW MAY WE CHECK THIS REFERENCE

APPLICANT'S AFFIDAVIT:

I CERTIFY THAT THE INFORMATION CONTAINED IN THIS APPLICATION IS CORRECT TO THE BEST OF MY KNOWLEDGE. I AUTHORIZE INVESTIGATION OF ALL MATTERS CONTAINED IN THIS APPLICATION AND AGREE THAT ANY MISLEADING OR FALSE STATEMENTS WOULD BE CAUSE FOR REJECTION OF THIS APPLICATION OR WOULD BE SUFFICIENT CAUSE FOR DISMISSAL AFTER MY EMPLOYMENT. I UNDERSTAND THAT MY EMPLOYMENT IS CONTINGENT UPON SATISFACTORY COMPLETION OF A PHYSICAL EXAMINATION BY A MOUNT SINAI EMPLOYEE HEALTH SERVICE PHYSICIAN; THE RECEIPT BY MOUNT SINAI OF SATISFACTORY WORK REFERENCES AND MY SATISFACTORY COMPLETION OF THE PROBATIONARY PERIOD OF EMPLOYMENT FOR MY POSITION. I HEREBY AUTHORIZE MY PRESENT/PAST EMPLOYERS TO FURNISH MOUNT SINAI WITH THEIR RECORDS OF SERVICE. I AGREE IF EMPLOYED TO SUPPLY MOUNT SINAI WITH SUCH VERIFICATIONS AS THEY MAY BE PERMITTED BY FEDERAL STATE, AND MUNICIPLE CODES AND REGULATIONS TO REQUEST OF ME AND TO ABIDE BY ALL MOUNT SINAI'S RULES AND REGULATIONS.

_____   _____

DATE   SIGNATURE

Exhibit 3 *(Cont'd)*

REFERRAL:

DEPARTMENT NAME _____ DEPARTMENT HEAD _____

POSITION _____ REPLACING _____

PERMANENT _____ TEMPORARY: FROM _____   TO _____

RECOMMENDED SALARY _____ PRE-EMPLOYMENT PHYSICAL DATE _____ STARTING DATE_____

    **(SALARY RECOMMENDATIONS ABOVE MINIMUM MAY NOT BE COMMUNICATED TO APPLICANT UNLESS APPROVED
    BY PERSONNEL)**

ACCEPTED _____ REJECTED   (STATE REASONS BELOW)_____

SIGNATURE _____ DATE:_____

DEPARTMENT COMMENTS:

PERSONNEL COMMENTS-CHECK LIST-

and distinguished from the application blank. Only applicants who are hired should complete permanent records.

The Interview

The most valuable single device used in the selection process is the face-to-face interview. The employment interview has the following function and objectives:

> Employment interviewing is the open exchange of information between persons of acknowledged unequal status for a mutually agreed upon purpose, conducted in a manner that elicits, clarifies, organizes, or synthesizes the information to affect positively or negatively the attitudes, judgments, actions or opinions of the participants thereby making possible an objective and rational evaluation of the appropriateness of an employee for a specific job.[8]

While application forms are often sketchy, incomplete and at times misleading, the task of evaluating applicants, a most difficult and demanding one, is best accomplished through sound interviewing techniques. Such techniques require complex skills such as psychological sophistication, understanding of the dynamics of human development and familiarity with the kinds of abilities, motivations, interests and personality patterns best suited to specific work situations.[9]

The interview has been described as "the conversation with a purpose." There are four objectives of the selection interview:

1. Matching people with jobs.

2. Serving as a means for creating good feeling toward the institution.

3. Dispensing job and institutional information in order to provide the applicant with a factual basis for accepting or rejecting employment if offered.

4. Providing the interviewer with an opportunity for obtaining data relevant to making a sound employment decision, such data not being available from other sources. The selection of a truly qualified interviewer is essential to the success of the employment program. The successful employment interviewer knows in advance the kinds of information he wishes to obtain. Although he has a plan for the interview, he does not stereotype his interviews. Before asking the applicant into the interviewing room, he will have reviewed all pertinent information such as the job description, the job specification and the application form. He must schedule the interview so that enough time is provided to effectively draw out the applicant and provide information for both parties to the interview to make a sound decision as to employment. Enough time must be scheduled to ensure that maximum success is derived from the interview. In a study made by Man-

dell, the median length of total interviewing time per applicant among those firms participating was found to be 30 minutes for plant employees, 45 minutes for office employees, 90 minutes for college graduates, two hours for salesmen and engineers and three hours for supervisors and executives.[10]

In the case where a great number of applicants apply for the same position, it is important to conduct a screening rapidly to save the institution's time as well as the applicant's. Yet it is desirable to leave the applicant feeling that his candidacy has been given reasonable consideration. One of the most important steps in expediting the *screening interview* is to plan in advance those elements in a candidate's qualifications which are most crucial in determining his possible suitability for the opening at hand. For example, frequently it is a practice in the screening interview for the interviewer to spend a great deal of time determining the employee's technical qualifications for the job. However, the nature of the position may require the employee to work overtime or to work unusual hours. If the interviewer spends half an hour determining the potential employee's technical knowledge and experience and then finds that he is unwilling to work the required hours, he has wasted valuable time. The screening interview is merely an opportunity to determine in a rather general way whether the employee is qualified and suitable for the job opening. Intensive consideration of his technical qualifications and personality considerations should be left for the later stages of the interview or, if possible, for a second interview which might be called the *placement interview*. Thus, in preplanning for the interview, the interviewer should have isolated those factors which are essential for more thorough consideration of the candidate. For example, a secretarial job specification may have shown that the following qualifications are essential:

> Must have at least two years experience. Must be familiar with office routines. Must be able to type 50 words per minute and take shorthand at the rate of 110 words per minute.

Therefore, the primary objective in the screening interview is to put the candidate at ease and determine as rapidly as possible if he or she meets these *basic* requirements. The interviewer may then want to dig more deeply into specific experience, work attitudes and personality factors.

The initial screening interview indicates whether the candidate is generally qualified for the job. The purpose of the placement interview is to determine specifically and in depth whether the candidate meets the detailed requirements of the job and whether his work habits, attitude and personality are compatible for work in the organization. In addition, during the placement interview, the interviewer should cover every item on the application form to ascertain that he understands the candidate's work record and can verify (through questioning, reference checks and personal contacts) the data given by the candidate. Briefly, some of the basic areas to consider in following the application form during the placement interview are as follows.

1. *Work history:* In many instances applicants unintentionally (and occasionally, purposely) leave gaps in their work history or overestimate the length of time spent in a particular job. Sometimes it helps to verify information by asking the specific dates when the applicant started with previous employers and the specific dates he left. All intervening periods between jobs should be accounted for. The exact title or position description of each job should be clearly identified. Determine the specific title the applicant actually carried in the job and the exact, detailed nature of his duties. In each instance the interviewer should find out why the applicant left his previous employer. The interviewer should delve into the applicant's feelings about his previous supervisor and determine what the applicant liked best and least about his previous jobs. Very often attitudes or patterns of behavior are disclosed that are useful in evaluating his suitability for the present opening. For example, the candidate may show that he likes jobs in which he is closely supervised and receives a great deal of instruction. If he is applying for a job requiring independent action and general supervision, it may not be an ideal situation for him.

2. *Educational background:* An individual's feelings and reactions concerning his learning and educational experiences can often yield additional information about his job attitude. The interviewer should determine why the applicant left school (if he did), which subjects he liked best and why, and which subjects he liked least and why. He should check closely any unexplained gaps in educational experience.

3. *Outside activities:* Discussion of educational experiences often leads easily into discussion of other interests, hobbies and off-the-job activities. The interviewer should again apply the open interviewing technique and give the applicant a chance to talk freely about his interests and activities. If the job demands mental alertness, professional skill and curiosity, the interviewer should look particularly for interest in books, periodicals and technical journals. In listening to the applicant talk about his social activities, the interviewer should watch for clues which indicate the applicant's desire to associate with others or his interest in exerting leadership in group situations.[11]

Five Parts of the Interview

The interview logically breaks down into five separate but, in some ways, overlapping phases:

1. Warm-up stage.
2. Getting the applicant to talk stage.
3. The drawing-out stage.
4. Information stage.
5. Forming an opinion stage.

In the *warm-up stage,* the interviewer attempts to develop rapport with the applicant. It is important that the interview be held in uninterrupted privacy in order to develop a closer relationship with the interviewee. Almost all applicants are nervous during the interviewing stage. The obvious need to discuss personal information in an interview mandates complete privacy. There is nothing more disconcerting to an applicant than having his train of thought disturbed by an incoming telephone call or a third party entering the interviewing room and holding a discussion with the interviewer. Informality is an important adjunct to this getting-acquainted stage. Some interviewers use a topic of general social interest to put the applicant at ease. No matter which method is used, the intent is to remove the initial tension experienced by an applicant when he first enters the interviewing room. It is essential that the interviewer set an environment conducive to the flow of relevant information. One authority points out that the interviewer will be more successful in breaking the ice and relaxing the candidate if he gets the candidate talking rather than carries the bulk of the conversation himself. He suggests that if the candidate is tense, the interviewer may want to prolong the small talk; if he appears to be at ease, he may want to shorten it.[12]

The second stage is *starting the applicant talking.* Here the application form can well assist the interviewer in selecting the one good question to trigger the applicant's flow of conversation. For example, an interviewer in observing the prior work record of the applicant may start this stage off by stating, "I see that you worked at Metropolitan Hospital for three years. Can you tell me about your job and what you did?" He then permits the applicant to talk and set the pace.

In the *drawing-out stage,* the interviewer attempts to elicit from the applicant answers to questions which were not developed by the applicant when he presented his background. The applicant may have left out details.

The interviewer cannot afford to permit such lapses regarding essential information.

In the *informational stage,* the interviewer now presents a picture of the institution and the specific job under discussion. Here he must present to the applicant all pertinent information and answer any questions the applicant may have. This can be a very crucial part of the interview since the questions posed by the applicant may reveal a great deal about his needs, his fears and his aspirations.

In the last stage of the interview, *an opinion must be formed.* This is often done by making notes after the applicant has left the office. Exhibit 4 (see page 145) is an example of an applicant evaluation form completed by interviewers at the end of the interview. Taking notes during the interview is to be discouraged; if absolutely necessary, minimized. It can be very disconcerting and disruptive to the interviewee.

Pitfalls of Interviewing

The key to the successful interview is the interviewer himself. Too often the interviewer falls into one of the many pitfalls producing an ineffective evaluation of the candidate and a poor result from the interview. Personal bias is not uncommon, be it favorable or unfavorable. The way an applicant dresses, the length of an applicant's hair, his speech mannerisms, his ethnic background—all may affect the interviewer's impression. It is important for the interviewer to be as objective as possible in order to reach a proper evaluation. *Personal bias has no place in the interviewing room.* Most of these biases are illegal as well as improper. The use of pseudoscience and myth, ridiculous at times, pops its ugly head into some interviews. Some people believe that there are criminal types—that certain physical characteristics denote reliability, accuracy, loyalty and honesty. These "natural" judgments of character are completely unreliable and have no place in the interview. Although appearance may be important for certain jobs, it cannot be used as a reliable guide to ascertain personality traits. Another pitfall is the stereotype interview. Interviewers should not allow themselves to fall into a comfortable routine, no matter what problems may be present in a specific interview. Some interviewees require a nondirective approach while others require far more guidance in the interview. The interviewer should be flexible in his approach and be aware of the personality and needs of the interviewee. Still another pitfall is the illusion of previous experience. Too many interviewers believe that in order to succeed at a job, the applicant must have had exactly the same type of experience in the past. This is unsubstantiated by facts.

The interviewer should not show by word or manner that he is critical of anything the applicant says or does. This can destroy his effectiveness. Interruptions by the interviewer should be kept to a minimum as long as the applicant is presenting information relevant to the final decision that must be made. Talking down to or above an applicant should be avoided. The interviewer should be sensitive to his own use of language, keeping in mind the educational and experiential background of the applicant. Inappropriate standards should not be applied since these may be too low or too high for the job. In either case selection based upon such false standards can result in poor placements. By using higher standards overqualified applicants may be hired, leading to turnover and discontentment in the job. By using lower standards applicants may be accepted who will require intensive training and produce a morale problem.

The halo effect is not uncommon in interviews. An interviewer may find something good or something bad in the applicant's background or presentation and, therefore, judge all his credentials on the basis of this one good or bad aspect. The question of note-taking referred to earlier is the subject of much debate among specialists in the field of interviewing. There is no debate over the need for brief notes following the interview, but most practitioners believe that note-taking can inhibit the applicant from presenting a free flow of information. It is best to limit the amount of note-taking by unobtrusively jotting down impressions without giving an indication of censure or concern over the specific information being recorded so as not to embarrass or inhibit the interviewee.

Pell directs the interviewer's attention to the framing of questions. He suggests: *Don't* ask questions that can be answered by "yes" or "no." This stifles information. Instead of asking, "Have you had any experience in budgeting?" say, "Tell me what you have done in budgeting." *Don't* put words in the applicant's mouth. Instead of "You have called on discount stores, haven't you?" ask "What discount stores have you called on?" *Don't* ask questions which are unrelated to your objectives. It might be interesting to follow through on certain tidbits of gossip that the applicant volunteers, but it rarely leads to pertinent information. *Do* ask questions which develop information as to the applicant's *experience* ("What were your responsibilities regarding the purchasing department?"), *knowledge* ("How do you feel about heavy travel?") and *motivation* ("Why do you wish to change jobs now?").[13]

The Successful Interview

To review the ingredients that will increase both the effectiveness of the interview and the chance of a proper placement, the following check list is offered:

1. The goal of interviewing is to match people with available jobs. In

order to do that, the interviewer must know what he is looking for and place in juxtaposition information on what the particular applicant can do.

2. Ad hoc interviewing produces ad hoc placements; the successful interview is based upon a plan which although formal is flexible.

3. Tools of the game are necessary in this as well as all management techniques. Therefore, good selection methods must start with the collection of facts such as:

a. the job specification;

b. the type of supervisor and style of supervision to be exerted on the successful applicant;

c. facts about the applicant.

4. The most successful way to preliminarily assemble the facts about the applicant is by use of an application form. This form should be as detailed as necessary and tailor-made to the specific needs of the institution. It is not uncommon to use several types of application forms for the various skill levels in the institution.

5. The key to successful interviewing is sympathetic listening. People talk to people whom they believe will listen to them. It is therefore necessary to ensure maximum privacy, expend uninterrupted attention and display an interest in what the applicant has to say.

6. Criticism has no place in the interviewing room. The interviewer should be receptive to all information offered by the applicant and should not disclose a critical attitude as to its content. The physical environment plays an important role in eliciting maximum information from the candidate and in reducing the tension with which most interviews begin.

7. The successful interviewer is aware of his own prejudices and should try to avoid their influence on judgments he is called upon to make during the selection interview.

8. Skills must be developed in how and when to close the interview, how and when to communicate rejection and how to evaluate the qualifications of candidates for employment.

Reference Checks

Almost as prevalent as the application blank in the selection procedure is the use of reference checks. Yet, although a large majority of institutions send out formal reference checks, many do not use the facts presented in response to such requests. It would appear that many institutions request the information to attempt to affect the honesty of the applicant's responses since it is felt that the mere implied suggestion of seeking reference checks will improve the quality of response as to its accuracy. There is, of course, a

Exhibit 4

APPLICANT EVALUATION FORM FOR INTERVIEWER

Name _____ Job considered for _____

Interviewer _____ Date _____

INSTRUCTIONS: Your rating of each factor should be reflected by placing a check ☑ above the position on the
scale that best reflects your evaluation.

1. PREVIOUS EXPERIENCE:

   Consider similar job duties, similar working conditions,
   same degree of supervision exercised and/or received.

Below Average	Average	Above Average

2. EDUCATION AND TRAINING:

   Consider formal education, major fields of study and
   specialized training received for the available position.

Below Average	Average	Above Average

3. MANNER AND APPEARANCE:

   Consider general appearance, speech, nervous mannerisms,
   self-confidence and aggressiveness.

Below Average	Average	Above Average

4. EMOTIONAL STABILITY AND MATURITY:

   Consider friction with former supervisors, relationships
   with peers, reasons for leaving job, job stability. Consider sense of responsibility, attitude towards work and
   towards family.

Below Average	Average	Above Average

5. SUPERVISORY POTENTIAL:

   Consider previous leadership experience. Consider degree of aggressiveness, self-confidence.

Below Average	Average	Above Average

   OVER-ALL RATING FOR SPECIFIC POSITION:

   Consider all the facts you have learned about the
   applicant, how well is he fitted for this job in comparison with other men doing this work in the firm
   or in comparison with your standards.

   ☐ Above Average

   ☐ Average

   ☐ Below Average

   ADDITIONAL COMMENTS:

☐ Hire   ☐ Do Not Hire   ☐ Hold Until_____   ☐ Refer to_____ great deal of skepticism as to the validity of information elicited from reference checks. Certainly most institutions discount letters of reference produced by the applicant and addressed to that universal someone, "To Whom It May Concern." To ensure the accuracy and sincerity of reference checks, they must be private and confidential. The most common technique of sending form letters or form cards to former employers has proved to be less effective than face-to-face interviews or telephone interviews of former employers. It would be an excellent policy for an institution to check the applicant's last employer by telephone, using the letter or card form for other employers.

Reference checks are often completed by personnel departments who have little contact with the applicant in question. To further ensure the validity of the reference, it is imperative to attempt to obtain the reference directly from the applicant's former immediate supervisor. Therefore, requests to former employers should be sent to the attention of the supervisor identified on the application blank.

Another factor which must be considered in attempting to evaluate the effectiveness of reference checks is the general reluctance of most individuals to put into writing anything derogatory about an individual who has worked for them. This is less of a problem in telephone checks and still less in face-to-face interviews with former employers. When more intensive checks of prospective applicants' backgrounds are required, such work can be accomplished through organizations specializing in preemployment background investigations. Some of these organizations are national in character and have resources throughout the country. Their agents make personal visits to former employers and neighbors. Their reports are objective and usually quite reliable.

Preemployment Physicals

Most health service institutions have no problem in accepting the need for physical and health standards that must be established for specific jobs. With the advent of new regulations guaranteeing safety factors, such standards are given prime consideration. The preemployment physical is a useful and important tool in determining the employability of an applicant. Such physicals should be as all-inclusive as possible, but certainly extensive enough to evaluate the physical conditions which appear to be required by the job specifications. The applicant turned down for physical reasons should be so informed. Such examinations should be given in advance of hire in order to obviate the expense, complexity and embarrassment of terminating a candidate within the first few days of employment on the basis of a physical defect which might affect his ability to do the job and which could have been predetermined.

Affirmative Action

Affirmative action is a term widely used in the area of recruitment, placement and employee relations in general to describe a policy whereby employers are required to make an extra effort to hire and promote those individuals considered to be in a protected class.[14] Under present law a protected class includes those individuals who have been the subject of past discrimination in hiring and promotion: Blacks, Asian Americans, American Indians, Spanish-surnamed Americans and women.[15] With final interpretations of various aspects of the laws involved in this complex area still pending, at best we can only present an overview of the statutes which affect recruitment, screening, interviewing and final selection of candidates for employment.

Equal employment opportunity is the law of the land, mandated by federal, state and local laws, presidential executive order and court decisions. The effectiveness of these laws has been questioned by those who review statistics which indicate greater levels of unemployment, nonemployment and underemployment for minorities and women. Income levels have been shown to be lower for those groups, and there is indication that a most pervasive discrimination today results from normal, often unintentional and seemingly neutral practices throughout the employment process.

A sample diagram of one type of employment process is provided by the Equal Employment Opportunity Commission (EEOC) (Exhibit 5). It indicates several phases where rejection is possible during the employment process. These then are the critical areas of concern in implementing an affirmative action program. The major areas of affirmative action legislation and sources of legal protection under Equal Employment Opportunity guidelines follow.

1. *The Civil Rights Act of 1866.* Following the Civil War, Congress sought to specify that the newly freed Blacks be accorded full equity with white citizens of the United States. The Civil Rights Act of 1866 was initially interpreted as applying only to governmental discrimination. However, subsequent court interpretations have held the Act to include private sector employees.

2. *Title VII of the Civil Rights Act of 1964, as amended by the Equal Employment Opportunity Act of 1972.* This Act applies to organizations engaged in industry affecting interstate commerce, employing 15 or more persons, and prohibits job discrimination based on race, color, religion, sex or national

LIBRARY ST. MARY'S COLLEGE

Exhibit 5

Employment Process

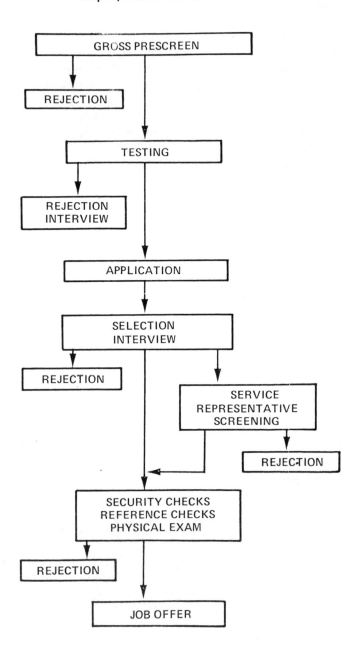

origin. The United States Equal Employment Opportunity Commission (EEOC) was created to administer Title VII and to assure equal treatment for all in employment. With the 1972 amendments, the EEOC is empowered to prosecute cases of alleged employment discrimination in federal courts and to order an employer, if found guilty, to undertake an affirmative action program to correct inequities. Title VII does not explicitly require affirmative action; however, EEOC has been guided by several court decisions which have remedial effects. When a court finds a violation of equal employment law, Title VII provides that it may "order such affirmative action as may be appropriate" for its elimination. As amended, Title VII now covers: (1) all private employers of 15 or more persons; (2) all educational institutions, public and private; (3) state and local governments; (4) public and private employment agencies; (5) labor unions with 15 or more members and (6) joint labor-management committees for apprenticeship and training. It is Title VII that defines the protected class categories consisting of the groups mentioned above. One major exception to Title VII is the bona fide occupational qualification (BFOQ) which allows an employer to hire employees on the basis of religion, sex or national origin in instances where religion, sex or national origin can be shown to be a bona fide occupational qualification reasonably necessary to the normal operation of the employee's business.[16] The other major exception is "business necessity" which allows the employer to disproportionately reject the members of a protected class as employees if by doing so he fulfills a specific business purpose or necessity that could not be fulfilled by any alternative employment practice. Courts have interpreted "business necessity" very narrowly, requiring overriding evidence that a discriminatory practice is "essential" to safe and efficient operation of the business and a showing of extreme adverse financial impact.

When a charge of discrimination is investigated by EEOC and reasonable cause is found, an attempt at conciliation is made. If this fails, EEOC may go to court to enforce the law. An individual, or an organization on behalf of an individual, who alleges discrimination may sue an employer and/or file a complaint with EEOC.[17]

3. *Executive Order 11246 (as amended by Executive Order 11375).* This order, issued by President Johnson in 1965, requires affirmative action programs by all federal contractors and subcontractors with 50 or more employees and contracts of $50,000 or more. Such employers must have an approved affirmative action program on file with the Office of Federal Contract Compliance Programs (OFCCP). The OFCCP has in turn delegated responsibilities to approximately 16 other executive branch agencies. Specific requirements for such "result oriented" programs are spelled out in

Revised Order No. 4 issued by OFCCP and are similar to court interpretations of Title VII requirements. In 1970, Order No. 4 specified 177 elements of the written plan and Order No. 14 stipulated how compliance reviews will be held.

Nondiscrimination requires an elimination of all existing discrimination factors whether overt or inadvertent. All employment policies and practices must be examined in order to establish a neutral personnel administration process. Affirmative action goes beyond lack of discrimination. In employment law, affirmative action means taking specific actions in recruitment, hiring and upgrading which are designed to eliminate the present effect of past discrimination. Minorities and women may already be qualified for better jobs, but continuing barriers throughout employment systems may be preventing advancement. The major part of an affirmative action program must be the recognition and removal of these barriers so that minorities and women can compete for jobs on an equal basis. The primary legal obligation of affirmative action is to change employment barriers which discriminate against people. The most important measure of an affirmative action program is its results.

4. *The Equal Pay Act of 1963 as amended by Education Amendments of 1972 (Section 6(d) of the Fair Labor Standards Act)*. This Act prohibits discrimination in wages by stipulating that equal pay be provided for men and women performing similar work. This is applicable to all employers having workers subject to a minimum wage under the Fair Labor Standards Act (FLSA). In 1972 this Act was extended beyond employees covered by FLSA to an estimated 15 million additional executive, administrative and professional employees, including academic administrative personnel and teachers in elementary and secondary schools, and to outside salespersons.[18]

5. *The Age Discrimination and Employment Act of 1967 as amended in September 1978*. This Act prohibits employers of 25 or more persons from discriminating because of age against persons who are 40 to 70 years of age in any area of employment. A major change in recruitment advertising has been effected because of the Act. Advertising copy can in no way imply age of a desirable applicant by using such phrases as "Junior Executive," "young," "retired person," "supplement your pension," "recent college graduate."[19]

6. *Vocational Rehabilitation Act of 1973*. This Act requires federal contractors and subcontractors with 50 or more employees and $50,000 or more in contracts to maintain an affirmative action program ensuring the hiring and promotion of qualified handicapped people. Section VII of the Act defines "handicapped individual." Section 503 requires federal contractors

to take affirmative action for such individuals. Section 504 forbids discrimination against the handicapped under any program or activity receiving federal financial assistance. The Department of Health, Education and Welfare published the handicapped regulations which implemented Section 504, effective June 3, 1977. Joseph Califano, Secretary of HEW, has said that regulations require "dramatic changes" and may impose "major burdens" on institutions receiving HEW funds.[20] Compliance with the regulations will require a revision of employment practices, provision of special aids and interpreters for handicapped persons and, in many cases, structural alterations to buildings. The statute provides: "No otherwise qualified handicapped individual in the United States . . . shall solely by reason of his handicap be excluded from the participation in, be denied the benefits of, or be subjected to discrimination under any program or activities receiving federally financed assistance."[21]

Included in the definition of handicapped are those suffering from emotional disturbances, alcoholism and drug addiction. Subpart B, Employment Practices, sets out requirements for nondiscrimination in employment of handicapped persons.[22]

7. *Vietnam Era Veterans Readjustment Act of 1974.* This Act requires affirmative action on behalf of disabled veterans and veterans of the Vietnam era by contractors holding federal contracts of $10,000 or more. Section 2014 covers regulations regarding employment of veterans in the federal sector. It is enforced by the Veterans Employment Service of the Department of Labor.

Implementation of Affirmative Action Programs

The mechanism by which an affirmative action program is developed follows.

1. *Workforce analysis.* The institution lists the total number of job incumbents from a protected class in each recognized job title within the organization. The numbers are converted to percentages known as "workforce statistics."

2. *Collection of availability statistics.* The institution must collect statistics covering each job title reflecting the number of available members of the protected class living in the organization's relevant recruitment area. These statistics are obtained from census information and other sources. Relevant recruitment areas, although usually defined by reasonable geographical bounds, can vary for different job titles. In some cases national figures must be used.

3. *Utilization analysis.* The institution compares its workforce statistics

with availability statistics to determine which job positions reflect underutilization of protected class members.

4. *Hiring and promotion goals.* The institution should identify areas of underutilization and prepare an affirmative action plan. This plan is kept on the premises and only submitted to the government if a compliance review has been initiated as a result of complaints received by the government. Annually the institution is required to submit an EEO-1 (workforce analysis) form.

5. *Penalties.* In some instances of flagrant underutilization the EEOC may require the organization either through voluntary conciliation agreement or by court order to pay money equal to the estimated losses suffered by the protected class members as a result of the institution's discriminatory hiring and promotion practices. The OFCCP is empowered to order similar cash awards through voluntary conciliation agreements, and in the absence of voluntary agreements to suspend or cancel the organization's contract.[23]

Conclusion

First impressions are lasting ones. The individuals responsible for recruitment in a hospital or home have far more responsibility than most administrators assume or are willing to admit. A substantial part of the applicant's impression of the institution is formed at the outset—when he first appears in the employment office. It is therefore essential that all employees assigned to the employment office of the personnel department effectively represent the institution: they must accurately and honestly communicate the hospital's policy and philosophy. In addition, successful recruiting is built upon successful interviewing techniques. A personnel director (employment interviewer) does not have to like people. He simply has to understand them.[24] Understanding people who apply at an institution's employment office encompasses the recognition of "uneasiness" and "concern" that the applicant brings into the interviewing milieu. Full recognition and appreciation must be given to the interview as a two-way communication vehicle: the applicant is given the opportunity—indeed, motivated—to present his full credentials to the interviewer; the institution, through the interviewer, is given the opportunity to present complete information about itself to the interviewee.

The appearance of the personnel office is the first indication of the institution's concern for people. The physical characteristics of all areas of the institution play an important part in molding employee impressions. The investment in a professional employment program is one that pays off in measurable ways to the institution. The cost of recruitment, often excessively high, can be minimized, turnover can be appreciably affected and controlled, and the institution can depend upon a pool of competent and qualified employees.

Notes

1. Arthur R. Pell, *Recruiting and Selecting Personnel* (New York: Regents Publishing Company, A Division of Simon and Schuster, 1969), Preface.

2. *Ibid.*, p. 42.

3. *Ibid.*, pp. 19-21.

4. Richard P. Calhoun, *Managing Personnel* (New York: Harper & Row, 1966), pp. 147-8.

5. Milton M. Mandell, *Choosing the Right Man for the Job* (New York: American Management Association, 1964), p. 158.

6. Lipsett, Rodgers, and Kentner, *Personnel Selection and Recruitment* (Boston: Allyn & Bacon, Inc., 1964), p. 42.

7. Mandell, *op. cit.,* p. 186.

8. Dean B. Peskin, *Human Behavior and Employment Interviewing* (New York: American Management Association, 1971), p. 12.

9. Theodore Hariton, *Interview: The Executive's Guide to Selecting the Right Personnel* (New York: Hastings House Publishers, 1971), p. 11.

10. Milton M. Mandell, *Employment Interview,* No. 47 (New York: American Management Association, 1961).

11. Material for this part of the chapter developed with the assistance of Dr. Leslie M. Slote, Management Consultant.

12. Hariton, *op. cit.,* p. 44.

13. Pell, *op. cit.,* p. 104.

14. James W. Higgins, "A Manager's Guide to the Equal Employment Opportunity Laws," *Personnel Journal,* Vol. 55, No. 8 (August, 1976), p. 410.

15. *Ibid.*, p. 407.

16. Eleanor Wagner, "Avoiding Illegal Employment Practices," *Hospitals, J.A.H.A.,* Vol. 49, No. 12 (June 16, 1975), p. 46.

17. For further information on Title VII, write: Office of Public Information, EEOC, 1800 "G" Street, N.W., Washington, D.C. 20506.

18. For information on the Equal Pay Act, write: Wage and Hour Division, Employment Standards Administration, U.S. Department of Labor, Washington, D.C. 20210.

19. *Ibid.*

20. Statement by Joseph Califano, Jr., Secretary of the Department of Health, Education and Welfare, Press release (April 29, 1977).

21. 29 *United States Code* @ 794.

22. Regulations Section 84.3(j) (page 22678) and analysis (pp. 22685-7), *Federal Register* (May 4, 1977).

23. The author wishes to acknowledge the research of Mary Louise Creedon, Affirmative Action Coordinator for The Mount Sinai Medical Center, and David Emerson, graduate student in Health Care Administration, Baruch College of the City University of New York.

24. Leonard Berlow, "How to Recruit Military Personnel for Health Areas," *Hospitals* (July 16, 1969), pp. 80-6.

ADDENDA

ADDENDUM A

How do the practices of the new renegade employment agencies compare with those of long-established, reputable personnel firms? Business Management consulted Nevin I. Gage, who operates a highly respected employment agency in Stamford, Ct. Here's how the two kinds of agencies shape up.

Service	Reputable Agencies	Questionable Agencies
Recruiting:	Engage in selective recuiting occasionally, and then only to fill the urgent needs of client companies at their specific requests. Most applicants obtained through newspaper advertising.	Do all their recruiting through a large, heavily indoctrinated staff of "counselors." Propects are called at home between 6 and 8 PM and Saturdays. This builds up reservoir of applicants. No selective recruiting for specific jobs.
Applicant motivation:	Encourage applicants to seek positions commensurate with their highest skills, to set salary requirements at high but realistic levels.	Promise salary advantages to raise recruitment volume. Later, urge applicants to reduce salary demands to to assure faster placements.
Resumes:	Always provide personnel managers with resumes whether requested or not. Encourage applicants to prepare detailed resumes in a professional manner. Help them revise their resumes when necessary.	Do not provide personnel managers with resumes if it can be avoided. Insist on blind interviews. Standard pretext: "We are selling you the man, not at employment record."
Screening applicants:	Interview in depth, to be certain that applicant is qualified in every particular for job he is seeking. Give approved tests when need is indicated. Question applicant to determine whether he is emotionally qualified for job and is likely to have a rapport with his prospective employer.	Spend minimum of time to get basic information. No testing by "counselors." Start here to maintain control of applicant and condition him to accept first job offer.

*Taken from an article entitled "Employment Agencies That Will Bilk You," *Business Management* (July 1968), p. 34.

ADDENDUM A *(Cont'd)*

Screening companies:	Study employers' record for fair employment practices. Do not send applicants to companies known to have poor reputations for job security, salaries or benefits.	None.
Placement follow-up:	After a reasonable interval, contact both applicant and his new employer to determine whether both are satisfied.	None.
Advertising:	Advertise only the existing job, not an imaginary opening so dramatized as to attract applicants.	None, or very little.
Counselors:	Employ only experienced, professional counselors with proved records for placing the right people in the right job.	No previous experience in personnel work is required. Persons with background in selling good or services are preferred. Persuasive telephone voice is an asset.
Job Orders:	Never send an applicant out for an interview unless a specific job order requesting a man with his qualifications has been received.	Rarely match applicants with job orders, except for general job category. Theory is that companies will be satisfied with applicants who approximate job description. Frequently try to "pump in" applicants.
Personnel managers:	Try to understand their problems. Don't demean them by attempts to reach department or division managers.	Regard company personnel managers as inefficient clerks. Try to bypass them whenever possible.
Fees:	Either make firm agreements with client companies so that the latter pay fees, or inform applicants that fees will be chargeable to them.	Tell applicants virtually all fees are company-paid, but have no firm, contractual agreements with companies. Applicants must sign contracts requiring them to pay the fees if they accept jobs and the companies refuse to pay.

158

ADDENDUM B

RECRUITMENT	Issued:
Page 1	Revised:

The responsibility for recruiting and screening applicants for employment rests with the Employment Section. The following statements describe the resources and methods utilized by the Employment staff and the guidelines that must be observed in attracting and referring candidates.

4.71 Employment Advertising: The Employment Section is budgeted and is responsible for the planning and placement of employment ads, selection of media and development of advertising programs.

    4.711 Individual departments are not authorized to place employment ads.

    4.712 In the interests of economy, a single ad will ordinarily be placed for two or more similar positions vacant at the same time in different departments.

    4.713 Although the Employment Section is responsible for the coordination of Medical Center-wide employment advertising, the suggestions of departmental supervisors are welcomed.

4.72 Private Employment Agencies: The Employment Section is responsible for the placement of job orders with private employment agencies and is budgetarily accountable for reimbursable agency fees upon the hiring of referred applicants.

    4.721 Individual departments are not authorized to deal directly with private employment agencies.

    4.722 The Employment Section determines whether a position is to be recruited through a private agency.

    4.723 The Employment Section selects the agency(s) based on such factors as ability to attract and screen qualified applicants, fee schedule, fee payment and refund arrangements, agency advertising practices, etc.

    4.724 The Employment Section determines whether an agency fee will be reimbursed by the Institution.

    4.725 The Institution will not evade nor abet an applicant or employee in the evasion of a legal obligation to an employment agency.

ADDENDUM C

PERSONNEL POLICY # 4.8	
SELECTION AND PLACEMENT Page 1	Issued: Revised:

The Employment Section recruits, screens and refers employment applicants for placement in vacant positions among the Medical Center's various departments. It is the individual department head's responsibility to select for employment the applicants qualified to perform the assigned work. The following statements describe the steps taken in the selection and placement of Institution employees, except professional medical staff, faculty, and social workers.

4.81 Employment Application: Employment applicants are to complete an employment application. Documents relating to age, citizenship, licensure, education, etc., may also be required. (See Personnel Policy #4.1, "Employment Standards"). Applications are screened by an Employment receptionist before an interview is held.

4.82 Employment Interview: Applicants meeting minimum job requirements are interviewed by an Employment interviewer. The interviewer elicits comprehensive information as appropriate.

4.83 Employment Tests: Employment testing is one of several techniques utilized in the selection of applicants. Test results are to be considered together with experience, background references, and the interviewer's evaluation as criteria for selection. Testing procedures are in conformity with Equal Employment Opportunity guidelines.

    4.831 Specialized employment tests given by operating departments are to be reviewed by the Employment Section to assure that test content is germane, administration is consistent and results are equitably applied.

    4.832 Test results, as all other employment information, are to be kept confidential within the Employment Section, and they are not to be disclosed to the applicant.

4.84 Reference Check: The Employment Section routinely checks employment and educational references, wherever possible, before a job offer is made. Reference check results are discussed with the departmental supervisor to assist him in making the selection decision. Unacceptable references generally preclude referral of an applicant to the department.

    4.841 Unacceptable references received after an applicant has begun work are discussed with the departmental supervisor

PERSONNEL POLICY # 4.8	
SELECTION AND PLACEMENT Page 2	Issued: Revised:

and, where appropriate, the Employee Relations Section, Security Department or Employee Health Service depending on the nature of the information received.

4.842 Discrepancies between the information on the application and the information obtained in the reference check are discussed directly with the employee. If the employee is unable to reconcile the discrepancies, the matter is brought to the attention of the departmental supervisor and the Employee Relations Section for resolution.

4.843 Reference information is confidential and should not be discussed with anyone, including the applicant except as in 4.842.

4.85 Departmental Interview: The Employment Section will refer to the department the best qualified applicants available. Applicants with less than minimal job requirements will not be referred. Departmental interviewers need not review with the applicant basic information elicited at the initial employment interview but should instead concentrate on assessing the applicant's specialized job qualifications in terms of the specific requirements of the job. The departmental interviewer should review with the applicant the duties, responsibilities and conditions of the position.

4.851 Before an offer is made, the departmental supervisor must confer with the Employment interviewer to discuss the applicant's acceptability, to determine whether additional follow up is required (e.g., references, licensure), to establish an offering salary, and to assure that appropriate pre-employment arrangements have been made. Job offers are made only through the Employment Section. Department supervisors are not authorized to make job offers.

4.86 Pre-employment Physical Examination: Before an applicant is accepted as an employee he must take a pre-employment physical examination and meet the health standards appropriate to his job assignment.

4.87 Licensure: In accordance with legal requirements and professional codes applicable to various professional and paramedical positions, the Institution will require satisfactory evidence of licensure, certi-

V. COMMUNICATIONS

> Effective cooperation in large teams requires purposive communication—
> that certain ideas must be shared among all teammates, and that informal
> communications cannot be depended on to achieve these results. Some
> essential ideas may not be communicated, while others may be circulated
> and modified in possibly erroneous form. Unplanned communication may
> have been adequate when working teams were small, when the whole team
> worked—and perhaps lived—in the home of the master craftsman, but such
> unplanned procedure cannot be depended on when teams include thou-
> sands of team members who may be scattered among the maze of divisions,
> departments, plants and buildings.[1]

Communication is the exchange—upward, downward, laterally—of
information and ideas. To be successful it must result in a common understanding between all who are part of the communication network. Much of
what the administrator or supervisor does in some way resembles what the
subordinate does. The key difference between the manager and the worker
is that the manager must get work done *through* other people. This can only
be accomplished by means of sound communication. Communication is
neither an appendage nor an afterthought in the organization's life-style. It
is the cornerstone of organizational life and existence. Within the complex
organizational patterns of the modern health services institution, it is clear
that communication programs must be developed on a sophisticated level
with the prime goal of optimizing understanding and effecting maximum
cooperation of all levels of staff. Of course, it is a *sine qua non* that communication grows best in a climate of trust and confidence. An administration
that does one thing and says another cannot in the final analysis expect
communications, whether formal or informal, to be effective. Still another
organizational life-style which is counterproductive to effective communications is referred to as "playing it close to the vest." Some institutions
believe that employees should be told as little as possible and that information should be disseminated only on a "need-to-know" basis. In a survey
among industrial workers conducted in the early 1950's (see Exhibit 1, page
164), employees indicated that "feeling in on things" was one of the major
needs not fulfilled by their management. Rounding out the three most
important needs expressed by these workers was "full appreciation of work

163

done" and "sympathetic help on personal problems."[2] It is readily seen from this study that the three major needs expressed by workers dealt with the communication patterns—too often guarded, meager or neglected—of the institution.

Exhibit 1

WHAT DO WORKERS WANT MOST?

The average foreman says that good wages, job security, and promotion are his workers' basic desires.

Workers rate full appreciation of work done, feeling "in" on things, and sympathetic help on personal problems as their chief wants. But foremen say these are the least of their workers' job goals.

These are the finding of a spot survey conducted by *FOREMAN FACTS* in 24 industrial plants. Foremen were asked to rank the 10 key factors listed below in the order of their importance to workers. Then workers in the same plant were asked to do the same. When the two lists were matched these were the results:

JOB GOAL	Ranked by Workers	Ranked by Foremen
Full apprecation of work done	1st	8th
Feeling "in" on things	2nd	10th
Sympathetic help on personal problems	3rd	9th
Job security	4th	2nd
Good wages	5th	1st
"Work that keeps you interested"	6th	5th
Promotion and growth in company	7th	3rd
Personal loyalty to workers	8th	6th
Good working conditions	9th	4th
Tactful disciplining	10th	7th

Source: Foreman Facts, Vol. 9, No. 21 (Newark, N.J.: Labor Relations Institute).

Drucker urges upon all institutions an improvement in general employee comunications. "To measure work against objectives requires information . . . Management must try to convey this information—not because the worker wants it, but because the best interest of the enterprise demands that he have it. The great mass of employees may never be reached even with the best of efforts, but only by trying to get information to every worker can management hope to reach the small group that in every plant, office or store leads public opinion and molds common attitudes."[3]

Planning Communication

The planning of communications is essential to producing the resultant optimum objectives. It is inconceivable to think of any form of interpersonal relationship and activity which is not dependent upon communication. One study found that the typical executive spends about 75 percent of his time communicating and about 75 percent of this time communicating in individual face-to-face situations.[4] Too often, even though the parties are speaking the same language, understanding escapes either one or the other. Merrihue suggests the following essential steps in the planning of communication:[5]

1. Know your objective. What is it that you intend to accomplish by this communication? The sharper the focus, the better the result.

2. Identify your audience. It is necessary to know who you are communicating with in order to select the proper language and the proper media.

3. Determine your medium (or media). The method of communication will often determine the success of the communication. A decision must be made on how best to communicate the message.

4. Tailor the communication to fit the relationship between sender and receiver. The key to this element of effective communication is the relationship climate. Is it one of fear or confidence?

5. Establish a mutuality of interest. Empathy, the ability to see the other person's point of view, is a priceless ingredient of effective communication.

6. Watch your timing. This is critical to the effectiveness of the communication. It is important to decide who should receive the communication first.

7. Measure results. Has the desired response occurred?

Essentials of Good Communication

It is a well-established principle that there is a positive relationship between good supervisory communication and effective performance. There are basic rules which are the cornerstone of successful communications:

1. Before communicating, clarify the idea in your mind. Too often we tend to communicate with undefined ideas and unclear objectives.

2. Examine the *real* objective of the communication. It is important to establish at the outset the goal or central reason for the communication.

3. Adapt the language of the communication and the setting to the specific situation. It is essential that the proper words be selected with regard to the intelligence and background of experience of the receiver. The total

physical and human setting must be considered in planning for effective communications. This includes a sense of timing and, of course, the physical setting which must afford both participants privacy, if necessary.

4. It is often not what you communicate but how you communicate that will effect results. It is imperative that the sender be sensitive to the importance of his tone of voice, expression and, of course, as mentioned before, his language.

5. Communication should be precise, brief and clear in presenting facts. Unnecessary words complicate communications. All facts should be stated in as objective terms as possible, avoiding abstractions and, whenever possible, providing illustrations.

6. Follow up communications. It is important to measure results to see how effective the communication was and, of course, learn from the mistakes of ineffective communicating.

Listening: The Key to Good Communication

Sitting *up* and listening is half (at least) of the process of communication. Developing the art of listening requires in most cases relearning and unlearning bad habits developed over the years. Most of us do not know how to listen. We are often guilty of listening for facts or listening intelligently for the verbal statement alone when the art of listening is the discerning of ideas. Our biases also enter into our listening habits. It is not unusual for certain words—rhetoric—to prejudice our appreciation and understanding. We may well not like the way a speaker "looks" or not like his voice and, therefore, pay little attention to or discount what he has to say. Some of the prevalent and counterproductive listening habits follow:

1. Talking too much. It is obvious that if one talks too much, one cannot have enough time to listen.

    a. Do you spend too much time explaining or defending your own position, thereby neglecting a careful evaluation of the other individual's position?

    b. Are you so intent on framing the answer to a question which has yet to be fully communicated to you that indeed you stop listening in the midst of someone's communication?

    c. Are you often puzzled about what the other individual really meant?

All of these actions require a reassessment of our "talking" and "listening" habits. The key to these problems is in disciplining oneself to ask questions and wait—remaining silent—for enough time to pass for the other individual to communicate to you. It requires a disciplined approach to listening by appreciating the power of silence.

2. Asking leading questions. One of the most common pitfalls of communication is framing questions in such a way that the "right answer" is obtained.

   a. Are you receiving only the answers you were secretly wishing for?

   b. Are you receiving only limited responses which are guarded?

In order to obtain the true responses of people to whom you are communicating, it would be best to outline the important areas in which questions should be asked and to frame the questions so that they are "open-ended." This will leave the other individual free to answer in any way and in as elaborate a fashion as he chooses.

3. Selecting the wrong time and the wrong place to communicate.

   a. Is your communication hasty and does it reflect your desire to hurry it?

   b. Do you have one foot out the door and only one ear unlocked when communicating?

   c. Do you communicate in public when the subject cries for a private audience?

   d. Are the phones ringing? Do people come barging in? Are you constantly distracted when in the midst of communication?

   e. Do you communicate too soon or too late?

It is best to plan your communication time so that a full disscussion can be had and the listener and speaker can give full attention to the discussion. It is also best to communicate in an atmosphere without distractions. It is important to be sensitive to the dignity of the listener; therefore, certain communications must be held in private and the listener should not be embarrassed in the presence of his peers.

A special study by the United Hospital Fund of New York lists underlying principles of effective employee-management communication:[6]

1. Communication should not be regarded as a tool or "helping" aspect of the organization, but as the essence of organized activity and the basic process out of which all other functions derive.

2. Communications should be subjected to accepted management principles of analyzing, planning, coordinating and evaluating.

3. Organizational communication should be thought of as directional—upward, downward or horizontally from the sender. Each direction poses different technical and psychological problems which must be solved if communication is to be successful.

4. Ineffective communication within an organizational system can mean wasted time and resources and, therefore, can result in lower productivity and higher costs than necessary.

5. It may be important to change an individual's attitudes—so that he

will be motivated to apply the principles and skills he has learned.

6. Although most communication is verbal, communication in a variety of nonverbal ways should be recognized: through gestures, facial expressions, body postures and movements, tone of voice and dress. Most of all we communicate by our actions.

7. People generally hear, read, observe and choose to understand only those parts of the message that relate to their own interests, desires and needs.

8. Our choice is not between communicating or not communicating, but between communicating effectively or ineffectively, between contributing or not contributing to reach the goals of the organization.

9. Repetition is important in communication. Many people miss a message the first time around.

10. Feedback is a critical element in communication. There must be a way for the sender to observe the effect of his message on the receiver's behavior.

11. The greatest barrier to communication probably lies in the area of human relationships.

12. Communication does not occur merely because the message is *sent;* it must also be *received* with reasonable fidelity.

13. The administrator should think not only of solving "communication" problems per se, but also of solving specific organizational problems by consciously applying specific communication techniques.

Insulated Chief Administrators

McMurry points out that many institutions, in spite of the expenditure of huge sums for communications programs, have top administrators who are totally—or almost totally—insulated from what is actually taking place in their own institution. It has been found that much of the information which reaches the chief executive is often incomplete and biased. This is not fortuitous, but rather reflects a temperamental disposition on the part of the chief executive which filters down the line and makes obvious that he (the chief administrator) is not able to accept and assimilate information which happens to conflict with his own values and predilections. There is a great deal of inaccuracy of information transmitted up the line. Add to this the many communication barriers and one would suspect a carefully designed attempt to filter information that reaches the chief administrator. According to McMurry, there are many reasons for this:[7]

1. No subordinate wishes to have his superior learn of anything he interprets to be actually or potentially discreditable to him. He therefore screens information and colors communication.

2. Subordinates soon learn what their superior desires to hear. The subordinate's personal anxieties, hostilities, aspirations and system of beliefs and values must inevitably shape and color his interpretation and acceptance of what he has learned and is expected to transmit.

3. Subordinates are often desirous of impressing their superior with the superiority of *their* contribution to the institution and, by the same token, of the inadequacies of the contribution of their rivals.

A chief administrator who wishes to obtain accurate information must develop an organizational style permeated by trust and confidence which will invite a free flow and exchange of information up and down the line.

Factors that Influence Meaning

Merrihue states that how much and how accurately meaning is conveyed in communication depends on a number of factors and lists the following:[8]

1. *The functional relationship between the sender and the receiver.* Very often they differ sharply in their policy thinking and their sense of values.

2. *The positional relationship between sender and receiver.* Is it that of an old-timer authoritatively instructing the newcomer? Is it that of a president speaking to a workman?

3. *The group membership relationship.* Is it that of management speaking to management or a member of a union which is overtly hostile to management?

4. Differences in heredity and prior environment. Are the backgrounds of sender and receiver relatively homogeneous? If not, meaning will be difficult to convey. Status in life powerfully shapes ideas and attitudes.

5. *Differences in formal education.* What is the capacity of the audience to understand and comprehend the message?

6. *Past experience.* What has been the quality of the human relationships between sender and receiver?

7. *Emotions.* The current emotional state of the sender and receiver can determine whether the correct meaning is exchanged or whether all meaning will be blocked by an insurmountable barrier.

8. *Misunderstanding of words (and the vagaries of semantics).* Words alone do not convey meaning. Only people can convey meaning through their use of words.

Communication has been likened to a radio set. First, you must select the station. The radio must be tuned for sending and the receiver must be tuned for reception. Selecting the station or the best wave length is critical. There are many messages involved in normal conversation, and often what the speaker means to say and what he actually says differ; in addition, what the other person hears is not always what the other person thinks he hears. In order to maximize communication skills and communicate what you intend to communicate, Odiorne offers a number of principles:[9]

1. Before sending a message, clarify your intentions quite clearly.

2. In shaping your intentions into language or "code," be certain it is couched in a language or code that the receiver will be able to manage with facility.

3. In transmitting, make certain that all of the media which exist as a channel of communication between the sender and the receiver are being exploited or at least sufficiently exploited so that the major portion of the message has a possibility of getting through to the receiver.

4. One of the basic requirements of good communication is that the sender have in his mind an accurate image of the receiver and of his decoded capacity.

5. This, of course, requires that he have an image of the receiver himself, his interests, endowments and attitudes toward the sender and the environment in which the message is taking place.

6. Good communications require that there be some interchange, back and forth, between the sender and the receiver in order that the normal, natural inconsistencies and lack of clarity between the sender and receiver in any message be made clear.

Communication Media

Hospitals and homes primarily make use of four methods of communication: meetings and conferences, hospital/home or departmental letters, written memoranda and bulletin boards.

Meetings and Conferences

Probably the most widely used method of communication is through meetings and conferences. A critical point in such vehicles is the ability for two-way communication. Conferences usually fall into a didactic pattern with all messages going one way. A conference that provides for discussion and encourages normal give-and-take can be most effective in the communication network. The truly effective conference involves a group of people pooling ideas and experiences. It is well to appreciate that the most effective conference develops from the acceptance of certain preconditions:

1. The meeting is called for a definite purpose, clearly understood by the chairman and participants.

2. The size of the group is limited.

3. Attention is given to the proper grouping of employee levels for the purpose clearly understood (see precondition 1, above).

4. The conference is of a definite length, and time of starting and ending is invariable.

5. A conference room should be large enough and comfortable enough.

6. Advance materials should be distributed to avoid time-consuming activities while the conference is on.

Hospital/Home or Departmental Letters

Letters sent from the institution or a department of the institution to employees are usually used in special circumstances. The announcement of long-range plans or of proposed changes are suitable subjects for such letters. To be successful they should be brief and careful attention directed to the language. This method was judged as one of the three most effective methods of communication in a survey of administrators.[10] Such letters are also used to welcome new employees, announce changes in employee wage scales and fringe benefits and in circumstances where the administrator or department head wishes to address a general appreciation to all employees. The cardinal rule here is that the institution should use such letters only when they have something of the utmost importance to communicate. Letters are probably the most personal of the communication vehicles. Most experts would agree that style is as important as content. Brevity, simplicity and a straightforward approach are all attributes of sound written communications. It is best to test the letter out on key administrators or supervisors before distributing it to employees. Careful attention should be directed toward common errors in written communications (see Exhibit 2).

Exhibit 2
Ingredients of Ineffective Written Communication
1. Subtle messages.
2. Limited interest subjects.
3. Rambling style.
4. Pedantic language.
5. Patronizing tone.
6. Incomplete explanation.
7. "Oversell."

Written Memoranda

Included in this category are the memoranda used between departments, between executives and between levels of employees. This form of communication has the advantage of permanence and verifiableness. It is often used to ensure follow-through between levels of supervision. The largest single criticism of this form of communication is that of wasted time and material: messages contained in memoranda can often be communicated, more effectively, by telephone. It is well to keep in mind that the written memo loses the most important attributes of oral communication— intonations and facial expressions. Brevity should be the hallmark of this form of communication. If action is required, such action should be clearly indicated along with the requested timing. Memoranda with hidden agenda are inappropriate. Directness and specificity are key ingredients of effective written memoranda. It is best to keep a copy of a memorandum that you have initiated, and good practice to send copies of your memoranda to any individual mentioned therein who may be affected by what you have communicated.

Bulletin Boards

Bulletin boards are an effective communication vehicle for formal announcements. They are most effective when they are able to attract employees by constant changes and careful control of content including prompt removal of out-of-date material. To obtain maximum efficiency from the use of bulletin boards, they should be placed near an entrance or exit, in locker rooms or in the departments themselves. Most institutions that make excellent use of bulletin boards agree that each department should have its own bulletin board. Two-section boards have been found to be the most efficient. One side is used for routine notices to the department while the other section is used for news items, special features, posters and general announcements of a personal nature. The use of posters is an effective and attractive way of getting the institution's message across. Posters may be used in formal series. Here again, constant change is necessary to keep the employee's attention. It is well to date all notices, first with the posting date and second with the date for removal.

Policy and Employee Manuals

An essential ingredient of a total communication network is the preparation and distribution of a personnel policy manual and an employee manual. Sound personnel administration encourages and facilitates the employee's optimum contribution toward and understanding of the objectives of the institution. The purpose of the personnel policy manual is to provide administrative and supervisory staff members with a complete documentary on the institution's personnel administration so that the policies and procedures approved by the institutions's board may be applied equitably, consistently and with authority. Personnel policies should be designed to promote the mutual understanding, respect and cooperation necessary to maximize the delivery of services in the institution. Exhibit 3 (see page 174) is a table of contents for a personnel policy manual. The institution must develop specific policies in the areas of employment, placement, promotions, compensation, benefits, training, counseling, disciplining, labor relations and many other facets of personnel administration.

The following are general statements contained in the introduction to a personnel policy manual.

Employment: The institution will use every reasonable means available to recruit the most capable employees for the positions to be filled. In compliance with civil rights legislation, and more importantly in observance of the institution's well-established tradition of fairness, equal opportunity will be given to applicants of all races, religions, national origins, cultural backgrounds, age groups, sexes and personal persuasions. Selection is based solely on the applicant's demonstrable ability and qualifications for the job.

Placement: The institution will make every effort to place employees in positions best suited to their abilities and career objectives.

Promotions: The institution will encourage employees to acquire the capabilities requisite for advancement. Equal opportunity will be given to all applicants for promotion. Candidates for promotion will be given preference over outside employment applicants wherever possible. Selection is based on the candidate's demonstrable ability and qualifications for the job. Where the ability of two or more candidates is relatively equal, the more senior employee is selected for promotion.

Compensation: The institution will maintain salaries competitive with those prevailing for comparable jobs in the health care institutions in our area. An equitable compensation structure will be maintained for the institution's numerous jobs based on relative responsibility, knowledge and skill requirements, working conditions and other characteristics. Employees not covered by collective bargaining agreements requiring fixed wages and increments will be given increases based upon individual performance.

Hours of Work: The institution renders around-the-clock service every day of the year. The scheduling of departmental work hours is based on the operational requirements of the institution. Employees will be assigned hours and shifts consistent with departmental needs and, insofar as possible, with individual preferences. Hours will be changed only with appropriate notice to affected employees.

Employee Benefits, Services and Activities: The institution will provide

Exhibit 3

PERSONNEL POLICY # 1.0		
		Issued: 11/1/70
INTRODUCTION	Page 2	Revised:

Organization

This manual is organized for convenient reference as follows:

Section 1   INTRODUCTION

Section 2   GENERAL PERSONNEL POLICY

Section 3   ORGANIZATION OF THE PERSONNEL FUNCTION

Section 4   EMPLOYMENT

Section 5   SENIORITY

Section 6   PROMOTIONS AND TRANSFERS

Section 7   COMPENSATION

Section 8   HOURS OF WORK AND TIME OFF

Section 9   EMPLOYEE BENEFITS, SERVICES AND ACTIVITIES

Section 10   PERSONNEL COMMUNICATIONS

Section 11   EMPLOYEE RECOGNITION

Section 12   TRAINING AND DEVELOPMENT

Section 13   EMPLOYEE PERFORMANCE REVIEW

Section 14   EMPLOYEE COUNSELING

Section 15   GRIEVANCE PROCEDURE

Section 16   DISCIPLINARY ACTION

Section 17   TERMINATION

Section 18   EMPLOYEE PUBLIC RELATIONS

Section 19   LABOR RELATIONS

Section 20   HEALTH, SAFETY, AND SECURITY

MOUNT SINAI MEDICAL CENTER

employee benefits, in the form of insurance coverage, pension program, etc., at least comparable to those offered in health services institutions in our area. Services such as employee health service, food service, group purchasing and personal counseling will be made available to improve the employee's working conditions and to assist in the fulfillment of his personal needs. The institution will also promote, support or maintain various programs of recreational or community activities to enhance the employee's leisure.

Training and Development: The institution will afford its employees every reasonable opportunity for advancement through increased knowledge, education, training and experience. Programs will be maintained for employee orientation, on-the-job training, upgrading training, tuition aid and supervisory and administrative development. Where appropriate the institution will provide educational assistance and training opportunities to members of the community.

Employee Performance Review: The institution will maintain programs for the systematic review of employee performance. Such reviews are to take place on a regular, periodic basis and the results of the reviews communicated to the employees. Supervisors are to supplement the formal reviews by keeping employees informed about their current performance progress.

Grievance Procedure: The institution will maintain a formal grievance procedure culminating in binding arbitration for the resolution of employee grievances. Every effort will be made to resolve grievances informally or at the lowest possible step of the procedure. No employee shall be discriminated against for having lodged a grievance.

Employee Discipline: The institution will pursue a policy of enlightened discipline, the primary objective of which is correction, not punishment. Supervisors are encouraged to administer disciplinary action that is equitable and in keeping with the offense; consistent with prior actions and with actions in other departments; progressively sterner after repeated offenses; and designed to persuade the offending employee to improve. Discharge is to be resorted to only if the offense is extreme or after every possible remedial effort has been made.

In a recent study, the following observations were made as to policy manuals used in hospitals:[11]

1. Very few manuals were readable. Generally they were verbose and poorly organized. Few manuals provided for easy replacement of old pages with revised ones; few had complete indices.

2. Administrators generally had no feedback on manuals—no way of knowing whether a policy or procedure had been read, understood or acted upon.

3. It is expensive and time-consuming to do a completely new manual, but one can be prepared and issued in installments.

4. Most administrators in hospitals and businesses who did not have policy or procedure manuals mentioned both the importance of such manuals and their lack of time to do them.

5. When policies and procedures have been generally understood and agreed upon, management may feel that there is no need for these policies and procedures to be written down.

Policy is a guide to action against which the administrator and the supervisor can measure his immediate, routine decisions that are often made under time pressure. Personnel policy is a simplification and logic-bringing instrument which assists in problem-solving and decision-making.[12]

The employee handbook is an offshoot of the personnel policy and procedure manual. It is more informal than its parent. Its intent is to explain as clearly as possible the policies and rules and general information of the institution. Many employee manuals are broken down into sections. The manual starts off with a welcome letter from the institution's chief executive. A section, "Getting Started," includes the organization's selection policy and deals with such varied subjects, necessary for proper induction of the new employee, as explanation of the probationary period, employee identification system and hours of work. Another section deals with compensation: how employees are paid, shift differentials, overtime practices and time records. Still another deals with important elements of "on the job" seniority, promotions and transfers and grievance procedure. A section, often quite large, will be set aside for time off. This will include an explanation of the institution's policies on holidays, vacations, sick leave, etc. The fringe benefit program is explained in another section. The obligations of the employee will be included in a separate section covering rules and regulations and general guidelines for cooperation. Employee manuals are often illustrated. Every attempt should be made to make them readable and understandable.

Assessing Employee Performance

The immediate supervisor or department head should evaluate the employee's performance at the end of the probationary period and at least once every year. The evaluation should be made in writing and discussed with the employee. Each performance review form is made a part of the employee's permanent employment record.

In considering employees for promotions or annual salary increases, supervisors should evaluate many factors such as skill, knowledge, seniority, dependability and interest in the work. Performance reviews play a decisive role in increasing career opportunities at the institution.[13]

It does not matter at which organization level an employee is: he (she) wants to know where he (she) has been, where he (she) is now and where he (she) is going. Every member of an organization wants to know exactly what the organization and, specifically, his boss expect him to do; how his performance will be measured; what his boss thinks of him; which areas need improvement; and how to move up in the organization. It is immaterial how well-adjusted an administrator is: almost all abhor the necessity to criticize a subordinate's work. Not only is it easier not to say anything, it is (paradoxically) even easier to terminate a subordinate's employment than to do the distasteful work of improving his performance. Crosby, in full recognition of the problem involved in assessing employee performance, stated, "Although most people agree with the general concept and purpose of formal employee performance appraisal programs, some express reservations regarding their usefulness and benefits. In some instances personal experience has caused people to doubt the validity of such programs. In other instances developing and implementing employee performance appraisal programs has resulted in disappointment. Unfortunately, these misgivings are used all too often as justification for total inaction in a personnel program that could help improve employee productivity, job satisfaction, compensation, stability and morale. A properly planned, developed and implemented employee performance appraisal program should preclude the possibility of failure and should prove most beneficial as a tool by which management can motivate its employees."[14]

Much of the controversy surrounding the evaluation process springs from the justification or lack of justification for the program. The key question here is: What will the program accomplish? There is little difference of opinion on the fact that with or without a formal program, administration will analyze and always has analyzed the performance of its employees. The appraisal function is a fundamental human act. Merrihue states, "The supervisor who obtains the best from his employees is the one who creates the best atmosphere or climate of approval within which his work group operates. He accomplishes this through the following methods:

1. He develops performance standards for his employees and sets them high to stretch the employees.

2. He measures performance against these standards.

3. He constantly commends above-par performance.

4. He always lets employees know when they have performed below par."[15]

It is clear from this description that the essential justification for employee assessment is *achievement:* personal and institutional. Mayfield insists that every supervisor should appraise his subordinates periodically and communicate his evaluation.[16] On the other hand, Odiorne writes, "I can see only mechanical policing methods to create and enforce the strictures of a deadening conformity. Individuality based on the capacity of each free man to express himself as a human being is not a value to be eradicated lightly and it should be cherished."[17]

Unfortunately the writers on both sides of the argument tend to deal lightly with the aspect of appraisal programs as part of an overall communication program. Is the appraisal program a means to conformity? Is it the basis for remedial action? Is it the yardstick to judge the next salary increment? Otherwise astute observers of the management scene have conjured up a phantasmagoria in the field of appraisals. They look at the mechanism too closely. One could find very little argument with their positions critical of the scales and ranking mechanisms, the list of personality traits, the impossible rush toward the arena of empirical judgment. On the other hand, one should not become enmeshed in the shortcomings of the means and lose sight of the worth of the ends. An appraisal program should aim at reinforcing performance by a systematic assessment of observable work achievements rather than intangible personality traits. It should be a tool for a plan for progress, not for conformity and not for criticism.

What Is Performance Assessment?

Performance assessment is a method of evaluating an employee's work performance on the job to which he is assigned. Other names for this method include merit rating, employee evaluation, performance review, performance rating, efficiency rating, personnel progress reports, employee rating and man rating. Wherever these names occur, they all mean the same thing: evaluating the employee's work performance. *Job evaluation* seeks to rate the value of the job with no regard to the performer; conversely, *performance assessment* or *merit rating* rates the person who actually performs the job.

Why Performance Assessment?

The assessment of employee performance is an essential management tool in evaluating employees for purposes of promotion, transfer, training needs and wage determination; in addition, it functions as a communication vehicle to bolster employee motivation and reduce counterproductive differences in conceptions of duties, priorities and accomplishments between the superior and the subordinate. Some administrators consider the employee performance review as a once-a-year administrative chore—a routine obligation that must be discharged in order to satisfy the personnel department. They consider the completion of the review form a tedious task and the conduct of the interview a superficial personnel ritual. Indeed, they find the communication of the results of the assessment embarrassing, distressing and without any redeeming virtues. More enlightened administrators view the assessment process as a golden opportunity to reinforce their relationship with the employee. They see it as a mechanism to provide support and guidance to the employee to ensure improved performance and development.

The primary purpose of the performance assessment is to *help the employee improve his job performance by:*

1. Developing and obtaining acceptance by the employee of the specific standards against which his performance will be measured.

2. Evaluating the employee's performance in terms of these standards.

3. Developing and following a plan of action to help him overcome obstacles to his development and to strengthen his capabilities.

4. Soliciting his reactions, resolving differences and reaching a mutual understanding of the implications of the review.

5. Offering constructive suggestions and tangible assistance to the employee toward his development.

In the final analysis, the question of whether an institution shall or shall not rate the people who work for it is an academic one. An institution has no real choice in this matter. Management *must* evaluate the performance of all employees. Judgments *must* be made and the only consideration is *how* to make them. Unquestionably an appraisal program can supply a yardstick to measure employees accurately. But who is to weigh the factors? Who, for instance, is to determine the factors that could accurately measure employee performance? It is the personnel director's responsibility to develop such a yardstick in consultation with representatives of the line administration. A program must be developed which will rate employees on the basis of an organized and systematic format which has as its cornerstone methodology incorporating common standards of judgment which can be applied uniformly by all raters. This is an essential ingredient since many performance assessment programs fall short of their mark because the factors being rated are interpreted quite differently by the different raters. Standardization of terms is a key to the successful assessment program.

Rating Systems

Performance assessment may be completed by one of several techniques.

1. *Assessment interview:* Here the supervisor meets with the employee

and discusses the employee's performance, offering an opportunity for response.

2. *Rating scales:* These scales are the graphic or multiple steps which require checking of an appropriate point along a scale of value.

3. *Employee comparison systems:* These systems do not require the use of an absolute standard; rather, the rater is asked to compare the individual employee with other employees being evaluated.

4. *Check lists:* This method provides an opportunity for the rater to indicate the employee's performance by entering checks in the various spaces provided (see Exhibit 4).

The last three methods involve the use of a formal rating system and may be augmented by a personal interview between the rater and the rated after the assessment is made. The *interview method* involves a face-to-face interview between the employer and the person rating him, and it is usually accompanied by a formal report of the discussion. The *rating scale method* provides for the employee to be rated against some "standard" that is defined or otherwise described on a scale. It is the most widely used method. Typically these scales are made up of five or more traits or characteristics. The most common characteristics are productivity, quality, job knowledge, versatility, dependability, initiative, appearance, personal relations and cooperation with management. In selecting the traits to be included on a performance evaluation form, there are certain basic considerations. One should choose traits that are:

1. Specific rather than general.
2. Definable in terms to be understood by all raters.
3. Common to as many employees as possible.
4. Observable in the day-to-day performance of employees.
5. Clearly distinguished from other traits.

The American Hospital Association, in its pamphlet *Employee Performance Appraisal Programs,* offers the following definitions for these most common elements in a rating scale:[18]

1. *Productivity:* (How much work is done consistently by the employee?) This element refers to the amount of productive work done by a given employee over a period of time. Depending upon the nature of the job, the output can be measured by the number of pieces produced (uniforms ironed, letters written, clinical laboratory determinations made), or it can be based on other measures (both good and bad) of quantity.

2. *Quality:* (How accurate, neat, or complete is the employee's work?) This element refers to the relative merit ("goodness" or "badness") of the employee's work. It refers to wastage; the effective use of supplies, equip-

Exhibit 4

THE MOUNT SINAI HOSPITAL

SUPERVISORY ANNUAL REVIEW

NAME_____TITLE_____CLASS_____

LIFE NO._____ DEPARTMENT_____

ADMINISTRATOR_____ TOTAL POINTS_____GROUP_____

DATE ISSUED_____ DATE DUE_____

INSTRUCTIONS — Read Carefully

Each employee's ability and fitness in his PRESENT occupation or for promotion may be appraised with a reasonable degree of accuracy and uniformity, through this rating report. The rating requires the appraisal of an employee in terms of his ACTUAL PERFORMANCE. It is essential, therefore, that snap judgment be replaced by careful analysis. Please follow these instructions carefully:

1. Use your own independent judgment.
2. Disregard your general impression of the employee and concentrate on one factor at a time.
3. Study carefully the definitions given for each trait and the specifications for each degree.
4. When rating an employee, call to mind instances that are typical of his work and way of acting. Do not be influenced by UNUSUAL CASES which are not typical.
5. Make your rating with the utmost care and thought; be sure that it represents a fair and square opinion. DO NOT ALLOW PERSONAL FEELINGS TO GOVERN YOUR RATING.

6. After you have rated the employee on all six traits, write under the heading "General Comments" on the back, any additional information about the employee which you feel has not been covered by the rating report, but which is essential to a fair appraisal.

7. Read all four specifications for Trait No. 1. After you have determined which specification most nearly fits the employee, place an X in the left square over it. If he does not quite measure up to the specification but is definitely better than the specification for the next lower degree, place an X in the right square. Repeat for each trait.

	TRAIT	S-1	S-2	S-3	S-4	S-5	S-6	S-7	S-8
1	**CONTROL** THIS TRAIT APPRAISES THE SUPERVISOR'S ABILITY TO CONTROL HIS OPERATIONS, REDUCE COSTS, AND INCREASE AND IMPROVE SERVICE.		THE SUPERVISOR HAS EXCELLENT CONTROLS AND CHECKS ON HIS OPERATIONS, COSTS, AND PERFORMANCE OF SUBORDINATES, RESULTING IN EFFICIENT AND TIMELY SERVICES.		THE SUPERVISOR MAINTAINS CONTROLS OVER HIS OPERATIONS, COSTS, AND PERFORMANCE OF SUBORDINATES, AND MANAGES TO PROVIDE ADEQUATE SERVICE UNDER UNUSUAL CIRCUMSTANCES.		THE SUPERVISOR MAINTAINS SOME CONTROLS OVER HIS OPERATIONS, COSTS, AND PERFORMANCE OF SUBORDINATES, BUT NEEDS OCCASIONAL CHECKING FROM ABOVE TO INSURE EFFICIENT SERVICE.		THE SUPERVISOR FAILS TO MAINTAIN ADEQUATE CONTROLS WHICH OFTEN RESULT IN POOR OR IMPROPER SERVICE AND EXCESSIVE COSTS.
2	**COOPERATION** THIS TRAIT APPRAISES THE INDIVIDUAL'S WILLINGNESS TO WORK HARMONIOUSLY WITH OTHERS TOWARD THE ACCOMPLISHMENT OF COMMON DUTIES AND COORDINATION OF VARIOUS ACTIVITIES.		THE INDIVIDUAL IS EXCEPTIONALLY COOPERATIVE AND GOES OUT OF HIS WAY TO COOPERATE AND COORDINATE HIS ACTIVITIES WITH OTHERS WITHOUT SACRIFICING STANDARDS OR POLICIES.		THE INDIVIDUAL IS COOPERATIVE AND WORKS HARMONIOUSLY WITH OTHER PEOPLE AND IS WILLING TO HELP OUT OTHER DEPARTMENTS.		THE INDIVIDUAL IS NOT EXCEPTIONALLY COOPERATIVE UNTIL THE NEED IS GREAT AND OCCASIONALLY INDULGES IN OBSTRUCTIVE ARGUMENTS.		THE INDIVIDUAL IS OFTEN DIFFICULT TO DEAL WITH. THINKS OF OWN DEPARTMENT OR UNIT ONLY, AND IS OBSTRUCTIVE.
3	**METHODS** THIS TRAIT APPRAISES THE ABILITY OF THE SUPERVISOR TO DEVELOP AND INSTALL NEW METHODS AND PROCEDURES.		THE SUPERVISOR HAS A BRILLIANT AND KEEN MIND FOR DEVELOPING MORE EFFECTIVE METHODS AND PROCEDURES, AND HAS AN EAGERNESS TO LEARN AND APPLY KNOWLEDGE.		THE SUPERVISOR IS QUICK TO GRASP NEW IDEAS AND METHODS, AND DEVELOPS HIS SHARE OF NEW METHODS AND PROCEDURES.		THE SUPERVISOR LEARNS NEW METHODS AND PROCEDURES SATISFACTORILY, SELDOM DEVELOPS MORE EFFECTIVE METHODS OR PROCEDURES ON OWN.		THE SUPERVISOR LEARNS NEW METHODS AND PROCEDURES ONLY BY EXCESSIVE REPITITION, AND NEEDS CONSTANT GUIDANCE IN IMPROVING OPERATIONS.
4	**PERSONNEL DEVELOPMENT** THIS TRAIT APPRAISES THE INDIVIDUALS FACULTY FOR SELECTING THE RIGHT PERSONNEL TO FIT JOB REQUIREMENTS, TRAIN SUBORDINATES, AND AROUSE THEIR INTEREST AND AMBITION.		THE INDIVIDUAL HAS A KEEN ABILITY TO SELECT AND DEVELOP KEY SUBORDINATES AND IS AN OUTSTANDING TRAINER AND COUNSELLOR.		THE INDIVIDUAL APPRAISES PERSONNEL RATHER ACCURATELY AND DOES A GOOD JOB OF TRAINING AND COUNSELLING.		THE INDIVIDUAL IS A FAIR JUDGE OF PEOPLE AND JOB REQUIREMENTS. BUT SOMETIMES DOES NOT DO A GOOD JOB OF TRAINING AND COUNSELLING.		THE INDIVIDUAL IS A POOR JUDGE OF PEOPLE AND JOB REQUIREMENTS AND HAS POOR TRAINING ABILITY.
5	**PLANNING AND ORGANIZING** THIS TRAIT APPRAISES THE INDIVIDUAL'S ABILITY TO ORGANIZE, PLAN AND DELEGATE THE WORK FOR WHICH HE IS RESPONSIBLE.		THE SUPERVISOR DOES FIRST THINGS FIRST, CORRECTLY EVALUATES WHAT CAN AND SHOULD BE DELEGATED, AND SHIFTS AUTHORITY AS WELL AS RESPONSIBILITY WISELY AND EFFECTIVELY.		THE SUPERVISOR GETS THINGS DONE. IS SUCCESSFUL IN APPORTIONING WORK LOAD. USUALLY ATTEMPTS TO DELEGATE RESPONSIBILITY AND AUTHORITY TO QUALIFIED SUBORDINATES.		THE SUPERVISOR ORDINARILY GETS THINGS DONE. BUT OFTEN FAILS TO RECOGNIZE ABILITY IN OTHERS AND DELEGATE AUTHORITY AND RESPONSIBILITY.		THE SUPERVISOR FREQUENTLY LACKS TIME FOR IMPORTANT MATTERS. IS CONFUSED WITH DETAILS, AND ATTEMPTS TO DO IT ALL HIMSELF.
6	**RESPONSIBILITY** THIS TRAIT APPRAISES THE INITIATIVE OF THE SUPERVISOR TO ASSUME RESPONSIBILITY IN KEEPING WITH GOOD JUDGMENT.		THE SUPERVISOR IS ANXIOUS TO ASSUME MORE THAN HIS SHARE OF RESPONSIBILITIES IN KEEPING WITH GOOD JUDGMENT AND COMMON SENSE.		THE SUPERVISOR ASSUMES RESPONSIBILITY IN KEEPING WITH GOOD JUDGMENT.		THE SUPERVISOR ASSUMES RESPONSIBILITY ONLY ON MATTERS IN WHICH HE IS WELL VERSED.		THE SUPERVISOR SELDOM ASSUMES RESPONSIBILITY OR ELSE ASSUMES RESPONSIBILITY WITHOUT THE NECESSARY QUALIFICATIONS.

▶ The reverse side of this form has space for general comments. The person making the rating is asked what he thinks are the supervisor's principal strengths and weaknesses, whether the supervisor might be more effective in some other work, and what further training might make him more valuable to the hospital. There is also a blank for a brief record of the interview at which the report was discussed with the employee.

ment, and materials; and the meeting of specified acceptable standards. It should not be confused with job knowledge, which is concerned with understanding, nor with productivity, which refers to the quantity of production.

3. *Job knowledge:* (How well does the employee understand his job assignment?) This element refers to the employee's job know-how. It refers to whether he has the necessary skills for his job and whether he can recognize defects in his work. It attempts to show if he knows how to meet the duties of his job, whether or not he acts accordingly.

4. *Versatility:* (Does the employee demonstrate ability to perform a variety of tasks?) This element refers to the mental and physical flexibility and adjustment necessary for satisfactory performance on a variety of jobs. It refers to the ability to change easily from one task to another.

5. *Dependability:* (How faithful is the employee in reporting to work and staying at his assigned work?) This element refers to the consistency with which an employee applies himself to his work, not to the amount of output or the quality of his work. It attempts to measure whether he works continuously. It refers to his attendance and punctuality; whether he remains at his job or wanders about; and whether he wastes time, loafs, or works in spurts.

6. *Initiative:* (How well does the employee begin an assignment without direction?) This element refers to the employee's willingness and ability to initiate tasks; to recognize the best way of doing them; and to follow up when necessary, with minimal supervision and direction.

7. *Appearance:* (Does the employee's personal appearance meet the standards for the job?) This element refers to the employee's personal grooming, attire, physical bearing, and taste. An employee's attire usually is dictated by the nature of his work, which should be considered in evaluating this element.

8. *Personal relationships:* (How well does the employee relate to fellow employees?) This element refers to the general pattern of social conduct demonstrated by the employee at his job. It refers to how well he gets along with fellow employees and may be related to such diverse areas as health, alcohol, family, and finances. Because this element represents a broad judgment of personality deviations from established norms, evaluators should rate it cautiously.

9. *Cooperation with management:* (Does the employee accept assignments and suggestions willingly?) This element refers to the employee's willingness to follow orders. It is related to his ability and desire to work with his supervisors as a team and to whether he resists or actively supports approved changes. It should not be confused with passive acceptance of orders or mere verbal "yessing" of supervisors to gain favor.

Frequently words or phrases are placed at various locations underneath the line of a rating scale for each trait to indicate different degrees of the trait. From three to five "levels" of the trait are usually so characterized including the two at the extremes. Points are assigned to various degrees of each trait together with a total point range for the trait. By adding together the points that the employee receives on each trait, a single point value—a total score—is deduced.

In employee comparison systems of performance assessment, the relative performance of various employees in a group is compared one against another. This method is sometimes referred to as the "Army Rating Scale." In such man-to-man comparisons, individual characteristics, rather than whole-man rating, are used. Each characteristic is described by five gradations. The high man and the low man are scored, and their names are put in appropriate positions on the scale. All other employees are compared with the names at the top and bottom of each trait to arrive at a rating. It is difficult to apply this method to the nonmilitary establishment since it is necessary for each rater to develop his own scale.

A modification of this method is described by Henry and Sparks. They discuss "alternation" ranking reports of present performance as a dependable method of assessing executive potential. The names of a group of employees known to several supervisors are listed on a form. Each supervisor selects the one whose present performance he considers *highest* and the one he considers *lowest*. Then he continues down the list to select the *next highest, next lowest*, until all are rated. He selects alternately until all names listed have been ranked. No specific guide of factors to be considered is used. Each ranker makes his own definition of what will put one man higher or lower than others on the list.[19]

Other types of employee comparisons seek to place all employees in a group in the order of relative performance, with best performance at the top and worst performance at the bottom. Some seek to force the distribution of any group of employees being rated into the lowest, 10 percent; the next lowest, 20 percent; the middle, 40 percent; the next, 20 percent; and the highest, 10 percent.

The check list type of rating offers a number of traits, and the rater merely checks the statements that best fit his assessment of the individual being rated. The list may be constructed with questions, statements, phrases or words which describe the manner in which an employee might perform on the job. The choice of statements is the key to the success of this plan; too often they are permeated with platitudes. Berkshire and Highland describe a variation on the check list technique: the forced-choice performance rating. This method offers a series of blocks of two or more behavior descriptions which appear to the rater to be approximately similar or equal in their level of favorableness or unfavorableness. Yet in studies conducted, certain replies are associated with certain levels of performance. An example of a block of behavior descriptions used for rating training skills follows:

1. Patient with slow learners.
2. Lectures with confidence.
3. Keeps interest and attention of class.
4. Acquaints classes with objectives for each lesson in advance.

A block of unfavorable items is:

1. Does not answer all questions to the satisfaction of students.
2. Does not use proper voice volume.
3. Supporting details are not relevant.

Prior studies have indicated that certain items can determine the differences between poor and good teachers while others have very little to do with the performance or relative success of the teacher.[20]

Developing Personnel Assessment Procedure

The key to designing a merit rating system is an evaluation of organizational needs. The system must be tailor-made to meet the needs of the organization. The steps in establishing a merit rating system include:

1. The determination of the traits to be rated. Usually the institution's administrative group will select traits which are specifically related to performance on the job.

2. Traits must be carefully defined so that each individual delegated the responsibility of assessing performance understands their meaning.

3. The traits selected must be broken down into "degrees" or "levels," and each degree, in turn, must be carefully defined.

4. The traits and degrees within the traits must be weighted. This process assigns point values to each trait which reflects the influence of that trait on the rating as a whole. The point values for degrees within each trait are established similarly by determining the amount of points for each degree of the trait.

5. The actual conducting of the rating. The employee's immediate supervisor should be responsible for the assessment of the employee's performance. This assessment should be reviewed by the department head and agreement arrived at between both levels of administration. Most successful assessment plans include the discussion of the rating with the employee once the assessment has been completed. Such assessment conferences include a frank discussion of the employee's accomplishments and weaknesses. The appraisal interview involves the interaction of two people, each with his own

purpose, knowledge, viewpoints and attitudes. While these differences may be difficult to reconcile, a well-managed assessment interview can help to determine goals and mutually acceptable standards. Both parties can then identify the problems that hinder achievement of their goals and arrive at workable solutions.

A constructive assessment interview is a very valuable management technique. It does, however, require the application of considerable skill, thought and effort. Workers want to know how they stand with their supervisors and it has been found that the whole assessment program is fruitless without a face-to-face communication of results, expectations and plans for improvement.

Administrative Appraisal

The assessment of employee performance does not stop with the blue-collar worker. Administrative appraisal is necessary to strengthen administrative performance by developing a clear-cut mutual agreement on work objectives, plans, and personal and institutional goals. Too often a discomforting situation develops by the absence of sharing the organization's total objectives by the chief executive with his immediate subordinates. The Mount Sinai Hospital, New York City, has developed an administrative appraisal program which incorporates three phases directed toward the final goal of sharing total objectives:

1. The personal appraisal.
2. The peer appraisal.
3. The supervisor appraisal.

A personal appraisal form is given to the executive whose performance is to be evaluated. The executive is asked to outline his job, describing the objectives, responsibilities and duties of the position as he understands them. He is then asked to list the phases of his work that he performs well and those he performs only adequately, and to make specific suggestions as to how he can improve. The narrative form of appraisal includes a statement on what he needs for improvement from his supervisor, from his fellow workers, from the organization and from himself. The executive is then asked to look back on the past year and describe what he considers were his chief accomplishments; to look to the future and describe the areas that he thinks he could profitably develop from the viewpoint of his personal goals and the institution's needs; and to list the changes he would suggest to accomplish such development. Concurrent with his self-evaluation, the executive's supervisor has selected one or two of the executive's peers and asked them to measure the effectiveness of his performance—specifically, to tell how well he functions regarding the needs of their department and how he strengthened or weakened their own efforts to perform effectively. They are asked to outline the executive's principal strengths and weaknesses. This peer appraisal is confidential and is shared only with the administrator's supervisor. It does not become part of the administrator's file. Finally, upon receiving the peer appraisal and the self-appraisal forms, the administrator's superior is asked to complete a two-part supervisor appraisal form based on the assumption that performance improves with coaching and self-development.

The first part of the form lists various phases of the administrator's responsibility: professional knowledge, willingness to assume responsibility, planning, controlling work flow and expenditures, and accomplishment. Here the supervisor is asked to measure the administrator's problem-solving abilities, report writing, meeting of deadlines; his organizational development and relations with the staff; his staff development and communications with subordinates and superiors. In each of these categories the supervisor is asked to identify which of four statements presented to him most accurately reflects the administrator's actual performance and then to support each of his ratings by briefly setting forth instances during the past year that demonstrate the administrator's performance in these areas. The second part asks the supervisor key questions about the administrator to be answered in narrative form. Among the questions are: What are his main strengths? In what respects is he least effective? What actions are you taking to help him improve his performance? Can you suggest any training or experience that will assist him in his development? This form then serves as the basis of the appraisal interview which is conducted in complete privacy. The interview aims not at criticism, but at improvement of performance through recognition of an administrator's strengths and weaknesses. The final step is to get mutual commitment to the goals of the institution. The self-appraisal section of this institution's administrative appraisal program is patterned after Douglas McGregor's suggestion that each subordinate should establish for himself short-range performance goals and ways in which he can improve his efficiency and that of his department.[21] (See Addendum F to this chapter for forms used in the appraisal program.)

Pitfalls of Rating

In making ratings there are several pitfalls which should be avoided:

1. Do not let your rating on one factor or your overall impression of the employee influence your rating of other factors.

2. Length of service or job classification should not affect the rating.

3. Do not let your personal bias enter into the ratings.

4. Do not be swayed by previous ratings.

5. Do not give the same rating on all factors (halo effect). There are wide differences in an individual with respect to the various factors. He might contribute very sound ideas and rate high in professional capability and still not meet schedules.

6. Do not rate on vague impressions.

7. Do not rate "sympathetically." If there are special circumstances, note them on an appropriate catchall section of the form.

8. Do not hesitate to go on record with your true opinion.

Ratings wherever possible should be made from accurate data or from observation. Ratings should be based on employee performance during the entire period being reviewed. The rater should be careful not to emphasize recent happenings or isolated dramatic happenings which are not characteristic performances. If an employee has had more than one supervisor during the rating period, each supervisor should complete a separate rating form. A composite rating can then be determined by the present supervisor. In the assessment interview, it is imperative that it be conducted in private. The employee should be permitted to read the review form, and an explanation of the supervisor's appraisal of the employee in terms of the requirements of the job—not in terms of the personal characteristics of the employee—should follow. Where possible, reference should be made to the position description or job outline. The employee's reactions should be solicited. The supervisor should listen attentively and actively. Criticism should be constructive and an emphasis placed on improvements to be made rather than on past failures. Unfavorable comparisons with other employees have no place in the assessment interview. If an employee's performance is deficient, it must be improved. He must be apprised of this fact. He must be told where he stands and agreement arrived at on future goals. The final step is the summary of the appraisal including the employee's strengths, areas for improvement, plans for effecting such improvement, assistance available to him and mutual commitment to the goals to be achieved during the coming review period.

Conclusion

The performance evaluation of health care employees is practical and necessary to ensure understanding and to obtain optimal agreement between worker and supervisor on the goals of the institution and the progress (or lack thereof) of the employee in reaching institutional and personal goals. A typical evaluation plan will be conducted as follows:

1. Rate employees in your department on one factor at a time.

2. Select the employee who excels in this one factor and give your rating.

3. Select the employee who should receive the lowest rating on that factor, and give your rating.

4. Consider the remaining employees, one at a time, and by comparison (forced choice) with the highest- and lowest-rated employees, determine the proper rating.

5. After rating all the employees in the group on one factor, follow the same procedure for each of the other factors.

6. After rating on all factors, review each form, taking into consideration the complete picture.

7. Ratings should be made from accurate data whenever possible, or from observation.

8. The rating should be based on the employee's performance during the entire period being reviewed. The rater should be careful not to overemphasize recent happenings or isolated dramatic happenings which are not characteristic performances.

Some change must be legislated if it is to be both permanent and positive. To ensure purposeful change, employee understanding must be obtained. This understanding includes the discovery of things the employee will both like and dislike: if change is to be effected, the worker must learn about both.

Communication is the focal point in a sound employee relations program. Studies in human behavior indicate a clear and urgent need for employees to know what is expected of them and where they stand in the organization. The development of formal communication programs is critical to successful administration. Too often employees of health care facilities, other than the medical staff, are the "invisible people." Medical staff and administration—that is, top administration—make decisions which are autocratically imposed upon the rest of the organization. Without appropriate participation and maximum communication, an organization may well fall below its expected goals. The hallmark of a sound communication program in a health care institution is the development and distribution of a personnel policy manual. Policies, plans and goals should be developed and communicated through various vehicles: conferences, meetings, face-to-face discussions. An organization that develops an atmosphere which facilitates and, indeed, encourages upward and downward communication will ensure its own success. Communication is not the responsibility of one department, i.e., the personnel department. It is not a "single-shot" program. Every member of the management team must be a good communicator. The supervisor's chief responsibility is getting the work done *through* other people. In order to accomplish this, a supervisor must be trained in the art of communication. This includes an appreciation of the importance of listening as an integral part of the entire process.

Finally, it is well to repeat: that communication grows best in a climate of trust and confidence is a *sine qua non*. An administration that does one thing and says another cannot in the final analysis expect communications, whether formal or informal, to be effective.

Notes

1. Dale Yoder, *Personnel Principles and Policies* (Englewood Cliffs, N.J.: Prentice-Hall, Inc., 1956), pp. 381-2.

2. *Foreman Facts*, Vol. 9, No. 21 (Newark, N.J.: Labor Relations Institute).

3. Peter Drucker, *The Practice of Management* (New York: Harper and Bros., 1954), pp. 306-7.

4. C. S. Goetzinger and M. A. Valentine, "Communication Channels, Media, Directional Flow and Attitudes in an Academic Community," *Journal of Communication* (March, 1961), pp. 23-6.

5. Willard V. Merrihue, *Managing by Communication* (New York: McGraw-Hill Co., Inc., 1960), pp. 23-4.

6. *Improving Employee-Management Communication in Hospitals: A Special Study in Management Practices and Problems* (New York: United Hospital Fund, Training Research and Special Studies Division, 1965), pp. 1-3 to 1-4.

7. Robert N. McMurry, "Clear Communications for Chief Executives" (special report published by *Harvard Business Review*, 1965), pp. 1-15.

8. Merrihue, *op. cit.*, pp. 18-20.

9. George S. Odiorne, *Personnel Policy: Issues and Practices* (Columbus, O., Charles E. Merrill Books, Inc., 1963), p. 103.

10. *Improving Employee-Management Communication in Hospitals, op. cit.*, p. 2-1.

11. *Ibid.*, p. 2-7.

12. Odiorne, *op. cit.*, p. 4.

13. Statement in *Personnel Policy Manual*, The Mount Sinai Hospital, New York City.

14. Edwin L. Crosby, M.D., Preface, *Employee Performance Appraisal Programs: Guidelines for Their Development and Implementation* (Chicago: American Hospital Association, 1971).

15. Merrihue, *op. cit.*, p. 122.

16. Harold Mayfield, "In Defense of Performance Appraisal," *Harvard Business Review*, Vol. 38, No. 2 (March-April, 1960), pp. 81-7.

17. Odiorne, "What's Wrong with Appraisal Systems," *op. cit.*, p. 79.

18. *Employee Performance Appraisal Programs, op. cit.*, pp. 7-8.

19. Edwin R. Henry and C. Paul Sparks, "Fueling Organizational Change at Jersey Standard," in *The Failure of Success*, edited by Alfred J. Marrow (AMACOM, A Division of American Management Association, New York, 1972), p. 296.

20. J. R. Berkshire and R. W. Highland, "Forced-Choice Performance Rating: A Methodological Study," *Personnel Psychology*, Vol. 6 (1953), pp. 355-78.

21. Douglas McGregor, "An Uneasy Look at Performance Appraisal," *Harvard Business Review* (May-June, 1957), p. 89.

ADDENDA

ADDENDUM A

INTRODUCTION*	Issued:
Page 1	Revised:

Purpose

Every medical center has four fundamental and interrelated responsibilities: to its patients, to the community it serves, to its students, and to its employees.

A medical center can effectively discharge its responsibilities to its patients, to its students and to its community only through the capable, harmonious, coordinated and efficient efforts of its employees. Sound personnel administration encourages and facilitates the employees' optimum contribution toward the objectives of the institution.

It is the purpose of this manual to provide administrative and supervisory staff members with a complete documentary on Institution personnel administration so that the policies and procedures contained herein may be applied equitably, consistently and with authority.

Application

If the observance of a policy or procedure results in a dispute or problem, or if the reader is uncertain of specific steps that must be taken, it is urged that the cognizant personnel administrator be consulted for assistance or interpretation. Compensation matters should be referred to the Wage and Salary Manager. Training matters should be referred to the Training and Development Manager. Employment matters should be referred to the Employment Manager. Benefit matters should be referred to the Benefits Manager. Employee and labor relations matters should be referred to the Employee Relations Manager. Matters having a broad or emergent impact on the administration of the Medical Center should be referred to the Vice President for Personnel or one of his assistants.

Changes and Additions

From time to time the contents of this manual will be revised or supplemented to reflect changed or new policies and procedures. Additional pages will be issued whenever such changes take place. The reader is urged to insert these pages as they are received so that this manual may be maintained as an up-to-date reference.

*Excerpts

193

ADDENDUM A *(Cont'd)*

PERSONNEL POLICY # 2.0

	Issued:
GENERAL PERSONNEL POLICY	
Page 1	Revised:

The policies in this manual define the responsibilities of the Institution's administrative and supervisory staff in relation to the employees of the Medical Center. These policies are designed to promote the mutual understanding, respect and cooperation necessary to enhance medical care, education and research.

The following personnely policy statements embrace a progressive employee relations philosophy to be shared and applied by the administrative and supervisory staff. They also provide the rationale for the specific policies and procedures outlined in the remainder of this manual.

2.1 <u>Employment</u>: The Institution will use every reasonable means available to recruit the most capable employees for the positions to be filled. In compliance with civil rights legislation, and more importantly, in observance of the Medical Center's well established tradition of fairness, equal opportunity will be given to applicants of all races, religions, national origins, cultural backgrounds, age groups, sexes and personal persuasions. Selection is based solely on the applicant's demonstrable ability and qualifications for the job.

2.2 <u>Placement</u>: The Institution will make every effort to place employees in positions best suited to their abilities and career objectives.

2.3 <u>Promotions</u>: ·The Institution will encourage employees to acquire the capabilities requisite for advancement. Equal opportunity (as in 2.1) will be given to all applicants for promotion. Candidates for promotion will be given preference over outside employment applicants whenever possible. Selection is based on the candidate's demonstrable ability and qualifications for the job. Where ability of two or more candidates is relatively equal, the most senior employee is selected for promotion.

2.4 <u>Compensation</u>: The Institution will maintain salaries competitive with those prevailing for comparable jobs in health care institutions in the Greater New York Area. An equitable compensation structure will be maintained for the Center's numerous jobs based on relative responsibility, knowledge and skill requirements, working conditions and other job characteristics. Employees not covered by collective bargaining agreements requiring fixed wages and increments will be given increases based upon individual performance.

PERSONNEL POLICY # 2.0	
GENERAL PERSONNEL POLICY Page 2	Issued: Revised:

2.5 Hours of Work: The Institution renders service around the clock, every day of the year. The scheduling of departmental work hours is based on the operational requirements of the Medical Center. Employees will be assigned hours and shifts consistent with departmental needs, and, insofar as possible, with individual preferences. Hours will be changed only with appropriate notice to affected employees.

2.6 Time Off: The Institution will provide time off -- in the form of vacation, holidays, sick leave, special leaves, and rest periods -- to give employees adequate opportunity for leisure, recuperation, civic duties and personal activities. The amount of time off and compensation therefore, will be comparable with prevailing practices in health care institutions in the Greater New York Area.

2.7 Employee Benefits, Services and Activities: The Institution will provide employee benefits -- in the form of insurance coverage, pension programs, etc. -- at least comparable to those offered in the Greater New New York health care community. Services, such as Employee Health Service, Food Service, Group Purchasing, and Personal Counseling, will be made available to improve the employee's working conditions and to assist in the fulfillment of his personal needs. The Institution will also promote, support or maintain various programs of recreational or community activities to enhance the employee's leisure.

2.8 Personnel Communications: The Institution will make every effort to communicate openly, promptly and accurately with supervisors and employees at every level. A keen responsiveness to improved communications will be encouraged.

2.9 Employee Recognition: The Institution will recognize each employee's individuality and dignity. Supervisory staff are to regard employees not as mere instruments of production or service, but as human beings with human feelings, human needs and human motivations. The Institution will maintain programs to recognize outstanding performance and long service. Supervisory staff are encouraged to recognize and reward outstanding employees not only through formal channels, but also in their personal interaction with these employees.

2.10 Training and Development: The Institution will afford its employees every reasonable opportunity for advancement through increased knowledge, education, training and experience. Programs will be maintained for employee orientation, on-the-job training, upgrading training,

PERSONNEL POLICY # 2.0		
GENERAL PERSONNEL POLICY	Issued:	
Page 3	Revised:	

tuition aid, supervisory and administrative development. Where appropriate, the Institution will provide educational assistance and training opportunities to members of the community.

2.11 Employee Performance Review: The Institution will maintain programs for the systematic review of employee performance. Such reviews are to take place on a regular, periodic basis and the results of the reviews communicated to the employees. Supervisors are to supplement the formal reviews by keeping employees informed about their current performance progress.

2.12 Employee Counseling: The Institution will maintain an Employee Counseling program to assist employees in dealing with personal, financial, legal and medical problems that may or may not affect their employment. Any information divulged by an employee in his use of this service will be kept in the strictest confidence.

2.13 Grievance Procedure: The Institution will maintain a formal grievance procedure, culminating in binding arbitration, for the resolution of employee grievances. Every effort will be made to resolve grievances informally or at the lowest possible step of the procedure. No employee shall be discriminated against for having lodged a grievance.

2.14 Employee Discipline: The Institution will pursue a policy of enlightened discipline the primary objective of which is correction, not punishment. Supervisors are encouraged to administer disciplinary action that is: equitable and in keeping with the offense; consistent with prior actions and with actions in other departments; progressively sterner after repeated offenses; and designed to persuade the offending employee to improve. Discharge is to be resorted to only if the offense is extreme or after every possible remedial effort has been made.

2.15 Employee-Public Relations: The Institution will encourage the development of courteous, tactful and considerate behavior among the employees so that their dealings with patients and the public will reflect a regard for human values as well as a respect for technical standards.

2.16 Labor Relations: The Institution will honor the right of employees to organize for purposes of collective bargaining and will abide by all legal requirements in this connection. The same labor standards will be observed for unorganized as for bargaining unit employees. The

PERSONNEL POLICY # 2.0		
GENERAL PERSONNEL POLICY	Issued:	
Page 4	Revised:	

Institution will join with other health care institutions for purposes of joint collective bargaining when it is in the best interests of the Medical Center and the ndustry. Administrative and supervisory staff should be fully conversant with the terms of our collective bargaining agreements and are to consult with the Employee Relations staff whenever a contract application or interpretation is uncertain. The Institution will observe all provisions of its collective bargaining agreements and expects the same from the employees and their representatives.

2.17 Safety: The Institution will maintain working conditions that are free of hazards to the health and safety of employees, patients and the public. To this end, a continuous safety program will be maintained with the active participation of employees, supervisors and administrative staff from various units of the Medical Center.

2.18 Security: The Institution will maintain security measures and provide the staff and facilities necessary to safeguard the property and personal safety of employees, patients and the public.

2.19 Health: The Institution will make every possible effort to promote the health of its employees by: maintaining an Employee Health Service; making available to employees its outpatient and inpatient services; providing medical and hospitalization insurance, as well as legally required insurance protection.

ADDENDUM B

GRIEVANCE PROCEDURE NON-BARGAINING UNIT Page 1	Issued: Revised:

15.1 Grievance Defined:

A grievance is defined as any dispute or complaint arising between an employee and the Medical Center.

    15.11 Greivance Procedure

        15.111 Step 1: The employee should take up the problem with his supervisor within a reasonable time. The employee will receive an answer within five (5) working days.

        15.112 Step 2: If the grievance is not settled in Step 1, the grievance may, within five (5) working days after the answer in Step 1, be presented to the department head or his designee. The grievance, at this time, shall be reduced to writing and signed by the grievant. As in Step 1, the employee shall receive a written answer within five (5) working days.

        15.113 Step 3: If the grievance is not settled in Step 2, the employee may present it to the Personnel Director or his designee. The employee will receive a written answer within five (5) working days.

    15.12 The non-union employee may have another non-union Medical Center employee represent him at any of the grievance procedure steps if he so desires.

    15.13 Should the grievance still remain unresolved after completion of Step 3, it may be referred by either the employee or the Medical Center to an outside arbitrator for an impartial and binding decision.

    15.14 Specified time limits are exclusive of Saturdays, Sundays and holidays.

    15.15 The costs of the arbitrator will be borne equally by the parties.

ADDENDUM B *(Cont'd)*

PERSONNEL POLICY # 15.2		
GRIEVANCE PROCEDURE BARGAINING UNIT Page 1	Issued:	
	Revised:	

15.2 Grievance Defined:

A grievance is defined as any dispute or complaint arising between an employee and the Medical Center.

15.21 Grievance Procedure

15.211 Step 1: Within a reasonable time (except as provided in the Collective Bargaining Agreement Article XXVIII, Discharge and Peanlties), an employee having a grievance and/or his Union delegate or other representatives shall take it up with his immediate supervisor. The Institution shall give its answer to the employee and/or his Union representative within five (5) working days after the presentation of the grievance in Step 1.

15.212 Step 2: If the grievance is not settled in Step 1, the grievance may, within five (5) working days after the answer in Step 1, be presented in Step 2. When grievances are presented in Step 2, they shall be reduced to writing, signed by the grievant and his Union representative, and presented to the grievant's department head or his designee. A grievance so presented in Step 2 shall be answered by the Institution in writing within five (5) working days after its presentation.

15.213 Step 3: If the grievance is not settled in Step 2, the grievance may, within five (5) working days after the answer in Step 2, be presented in Step 3. A grievance shall be presented in this step to the Personnel Director or Administrator of the Institution, or his designee; and he or his designee shall render a decision in writing within five (5) working days after the presentation of the grievance in this step.

15.22 Specified time limits are exclusive of Saturdays, Sundays and holidays.

ADDENDUM B *(Cont'd)*

GRIEVANCE PROCEDURE BARGAINING UNIT Page 2	Issued: Revised:

15.23 Should the grievance still remain unresolved after completion of Step 3, it may be referred by the Medical Center
to an outside arbitrator for an impartial and binding decision.

15.24 The costs of the arbitrator will be borne by the parties.

FORM L-08
3500 1-77 CAMELOT

THE MOUNT SINAI HOSPITAL
NEW YORK

PERSONNEL COPY

GRIEVANCE FORM

NAME OF EMPLOYEE _____ LIFE NO. _____

DEPARTMENT _____ DATE OF HIRE _____

JOB TITLE _____ DATE SUBMITTED _____

COMPLETE DETAILS OF GRIEVANCE: (INCLUDE SECTION OF AGREEMENT VIOLATED) _____

_____

_____

_____

_____

_____

_____

_____

_____

TIME LIMITS

(USE REVERSE SIDE IF NECESSARY)

REMEDY REQUESTED _____

_____

EMPLOYEE _____
(SIGNATURE)

DISPOSITION — STEP 1: _____

_____

_____

_____

SUPERVISOR _____ DATE COMMUNICATED _____ | ACCEPTED: ____ APPEALED ____
(SIGNATURE) | STEWARD _____

5 WORKING DAYS

DISPOSITION — STEP 2: _____

_____

_____

_____

DEPT. HEAD _____ DATE COMMUNICATED _____ | ACCEPTED: ____ APPEALED ____
(SIGNATURE) | STEWARD _____

5 WORKING DAYS

DISPOSITION — STEP 3: _____

_____

_____

_____

PERSONNEL DIRECTOR _____ DATE COMMUNICATED _____ | ACCEPTED: ____ APPEALED ____
(SIGNATURE) | CHIEF STEWARD _____

5 WORKING DAYS

ADDENDUM C

Listeners' Quiz

When taking part in an interview or group conference do you:

	Usually	Sometimes	Seldom
1. Prepare yourself physically by sitting facing the speaker, and making sure that you can hear?	_____	_____	_____
2. Watch the speaker as well as listen to him?	_____	_____	_____
3. Decide from the speaker's appearance and delivery whether or not what he has to say is worthwhile?	_____	_____	_____
4. Listen primarily for ideas and underlying feelings?	_____	_____	_____
5. Determine your own bias, if any, and try to allow for it?	_____	_____	_____
6. Keep your mind on what the speaker is saying?	_____	_____	_____
7. Interrupt immediately if you hear a statement you feel is wrong?	_____	_____	_____
8. Make sure before answering that you've taken in the other person's point of view?	_____	_____	_____
9. Try to have the last word?	_____	_____	_____
10. Make a conscious effort to evaluate the logic and credibility of what you hear?	_____	_____	_____

ADDENDUM D

COMMUNICATIONS MATERIALS
FOR A HOSPITAL.

Prepared by Albert N. Webster

October 25, 1966

*Reprinted with permission of the author.

IRCS
INDUSTRIAL
RELATIONS
COUNSELORS
•SERVICE
INC

GENERAL OBJECTIVES OF A COMMUNICATION PROGRAM

Communications with employees of the hospital shall support and be guided by the following objectives. These are designed with the intent of developing and then maintaining employee understanding and acceptance of overall hospital goals and motives, so that as a result employees will voluntarily contribute to the maximum extent of their individual capacities, and will cooperate as a group with the administration's steps to assure the success of the hospital.

1. To demonstrate the administration's concern and interest in employees as individuals--in their personal welfare and security.

2. To develop a concept in employees that each one's work is of importance to the overall accomplishments of the hospital.

3. To give employees an understanding and appreciation of hospital objectives, problems and results; to keep them informed as much as possible on matters that affect them; and to point out that their security is based on the sound, continuing and economical operations of the hospital, so that it can serve patients 24 hours a day and provide medical facilities for doctors at a cost patients can afford to pay, thus providing jobs, job opportunity and advancement of employee welfare.

4. To develop better understanding of management's role in the conduct of successful operations and the contribution of community resources in providing materials, machinery and jobs.

5. To develop and maintain employee confidence in the competence, alertness and long-range effectiveness of the administration, so that employees will have respect for (if not agreement with) the administration's operating objectives, programs and plans.

6. To convince employees of the sincerity of the administration's motives toward them, and the integrity and creditability of its policies and pronouncements. As related to union recognition and collective bargaining, to demonstrate to employees that the administration's position and goals are based on the balanced best interests of both the employees and the hospital.

7. To build mutual understanding, respect and confidence among employees at all levels and between organizational units.

8. To promote among employees the maximum possible regard for the hospital as an institution serving the interests of people and making an important contribution to the well-being of the community, and thus to evoke in employees a feeling of pride in the hospital as a good corporate citizen.

COMMUNICATION IS--

Behavior.......................... Speech, writing, action, non-
action, handshake, scowl, smile,
silence

that results .... Must actually happen, tested by
feedback

in an exchange.................... Mutual, sent and received,
listened to

of meaning....................... For both parties, related to needs
and/or interests of both

that produces action.............. Ranging from work or other desired
accomplishment to mere response
(agreement, disagreement, yes-
but)

SPECIFIC OBJECTIVES FOR COMMUNICATIONS AT
A HOSPITAL

1. To keep employees informed of current status of operations
and condition of the hospital

Maintain program of information to employees regarding
patient census, services rendered, areas served; point
out changes over past years and evidence of growth;

Discuss increasing costs, hospital's success in meeting
them, changes in methods, and how it keeps up with new
developments.

2. To gain acceptance by employees of the following objectives of
the hospital:

To make continuously available to the community the best
possible care of the sick and injured;

To employ a sufficient staff of qualified, satisfied employees
to provide the services required;

To protect the interests of employees as to salaries, hours,
benefits, working conditions, fair treatment, considerate
supervision, job security, personal growth, and to do so
without regard to race, creed or color;

To so manage the hospital that employees will regard it
as a good place to work.

3. To develop on the employee's part better understanding of his
job, and the requirements and standards of performance expected from
him

Develop and utilize organization charts, job descriptions,
performance standards and performance appraisals, and
discuss them with employees.

4. To give employees recognition for good performance

Assure salary administration based on performance.

"Counsel" employees for good performance as well as to
discipline for poor performance;

Arrange public personal recognition where warranted.

5. To give employees advance information on new services, procedures, operations, policies, etc.

> Explain the meaning of and reason for those management actions that affect their job or interests as employees.

6. To obtain reactions, suggestions and viewpoint of subordinate employees; to pinpoint problem areas

> Assure "feedback" of what employees are thinking, proper functioning of grievance procedure, and exit interviews;

> Encourage and take appropriate action with respect to employees' comments and suggestions.

7. To demonstrate that the hospital's approach to employee relations problems:

> Aims to deal with employees firmly but with fairness;

> Will seek solutions to problems in terms of maintaining a proper balance of the interests of patients, employees, doctors and the community;

> Will seek answers from all interests involved so as to assure the continued operation of the hospital on a sound financial basis.

8. To correct, answer or otherwise counteract inaccurate or misleading statements by union leaders, or distortions by them of management's statements or actions

> Monitor, catalog and evaluate misleading statements;

> Answer, correct, counteract or, by anticipation, offset the more damaging or significant statements;

> Select time (usually immediate), media and tone of communications most appropriate to give employees the facts, and develop understanding of hospital's intentions.

9. To improve communication skills of supervisors, managers and administration

> Define responsibility to communicate;

> Train by actual practice.

207

COMMUNICATIONS IN A HOSPITAL

The following communications have been listed by participants in Supervisory Development Programs conducted in hospitals. The list should be completed by the addition of communications used or needed in the particular department.

Columns are provided to evaluate each communication. Mark in each column:

1. More than adequate
2. Adequate
3. Needs improvement

The columns are for:

A. Manner--the kind, method, timeliness.

B. Substance--the quantity, quality, accuracy, etc., of the message or meaning being accumulated.

C. Feedback--the presence of an exchange between sender and receiver, opportunity to make contributions, talk back, disagree, ask questions, clarify.

MANAGEMENT RESPONSIBILITY FOR COMMUNICATIONS

Every member of management and supervision is responsible for communicating effectively with employees under his supervision, for ascertaining their reactions and opinions, and for communicating fully on pertinent matters with his superior and fellow supervisors.

Specifically, this charge imposes the following obligations on each manager and supervisor:

1. To give each subordinate an understanding of the work he is doing, the services he provides, and the reasons for the various demands made upon him in his day-to-day job.

2. When so authorized, to inform subordinate staff members promptly and authoritatively of all hospital policies and practices, regulations, objectives and plans, reasons, problems, successes and failures, and any other information concerning the hospital that affects their work, their individual status, and their attitude toward the hospital.

3. To seek out and use all opportunities to pass along hospital information and viewpoint, to be aware of reactions, ideas and viewpoints of subordinates, and to report information to immediate superiors, as appropriate.

4. To train and counsel subordinate supervisors in the use of effective communications and to facilitate the proper discharge of the responsibility for communications at succeeding lower levels.

5. To share information and experience across department lines as appropriate, and by so doing, to facilitate cooperation and coordination of joint activities.

It shall be the responsibility of members of upper management levels to specify in all management job descriptions the incumbent's duty to pass on information to subordinates; to appraise the overall performance of a subordinate member on the basis, among other factors, of his success as a communicator; and, finally, to demonstrate by their own actions that communicating is an inherent part of day-to-day management responsibility and thus set a pattern for those supervisors working under them.

It shall be the responsibility of the originator of a communication to determine, with appropriate staff advice as indicated, how widely the information is to be disseminated among employees. He shall indicate this in writing on the communication itself, for the guidance and instruction of those at lower management levels who will receive the communication and be responsible for passing it on.

	A	B	C
	Manner	Substance	Feedback
Oral, face-to-face or telephone			
Supervisor-employee			
Between departments			
Between employees in department			
Taking reports (nursing)			
Orientation			
Interviews:			
Hiring			
Appraisals			
Counseling			
Disciplinary			
Exit			
Public address system			
Training			
With patients			
With doctors			
Grievance procedure			
Expressions of attitude			
Social-recreational			
Grapevine			
Memoranda and other written media			
From administration			
From staff personnel			
From department head			
Job descriptions			
Policy manual			
Employees' handbook			
House organ			
Library			
Professional publications			
Procedure manuals			
Suggestion system			
Bulletin boards			
Patient orders			
Work forms (requisitions, orders, etc.)			
Reports			
Financial statements			
Tickler system			
Letters to employee			
Surveys			
Meetings			
Administrative conference			
Department heads			

	A Manner	B Substance	C Feedback
Meetings (continued)			
Within department			
All employees			
Special groups (head nurse, etc.)			
In service education			
Supervisory development program			
Trustees			
Ward conferences			
Open house			
Committees			
Inspections			
Medical staff			
Interdepartmental committees			
Departmental committees			
Safety			
Employee council			
Outside sources			
Medical forum			
Professional and technical associations			
Community organizations			
Vendors			
Schools-career programs			
Hospital speakers bureau			

ADDENDUM E

THE MOUNT SINAI MEDICAL CENTER
EMPLOYEE PERFORMANCE REVIEW

Name: _____ Position Title: _____ Life # _____

Department: _____ Date of Review: _____ Date of Hire: _____

Type of Review:
☐ Annual ☐ Promotion ☐ Other: _____
☐ Probationary ☐ Transfer

INSTRUCTIONS

1. Print or type all information requested.

2. Read through entire Review form so that you are thoroughly familiar with appraisal factors and questions.

3. Complete all applicable sections. Please be concise.

4. Write your evaluation comments just below the questions. If more space is required, please use a separate sheet of paper and number the comments according to the original format.

5. It is recommended that you dictate or write out your evaluation first and then have it typed on the attached form for retention in the Records Section of the Personnel Department.

6. The Appraisal Factors are as follows:

I. Job Knowledge	VI. Initiative
II. Quantity of Work	VII. Organizing Ability
III. Quality of Work	VIII. Development and Training
IV. Job Atitude	IX. Supervisory Ability
V. Judgment	

212

FACTORS FOR APPRAISAL:

I.   JOB KNOWLEDGE (Extent of employee's job information and comprehension) _____

    A.   Does employee's performance evidence sufficient basic training and experience for the job?

    B.   What type and/or how much additional training and/or experience is required for successful performance?

II. QUANTITY OF WORK (output volume, speed and consistency of output)

    A.   Describe employee's work performance volume and its impact on overall work quantity. _____

III. QUALITY OF WORK (accuracy, thoroughness, frequency of errors)

    A.   How well does this employee do work requiring thoroughness, follow-up and detail? _____

IV. JOB ATTITUDE (interest, motivation, enthusiasm and general willingness to perform)

    A.   Describe employee's relationships with colleagues, subordinates, supervisors, patients and visitors.

    B.   Is employee's job attitude consistent? _____

V.   JUDGMENT (extent to which decisions and actions are based on sound reasoning)

    A.   What types of decisions is employee expected to make?
       How effectively has this part of job responsibility been met?

213

B. How well does employee respond to <u>crisis</u>, <u>pressure</u> or <u>emergencies</u>? _____

_____ _____ _____

C. What are <u>areas of improvement</u> here and what steps are you and the employee taking? _____

_____

_____

I. INITIATIVE (creativity of ideas and actions, extent to which employee is a "self-starter" in meeting goals)

A. Give instances where employee has shown <u>initiative</u>. What were the results? _____

_____

_____

B. Does employee evidence <u>initiative after a problem is defined</u> or often <u>before a problem even exists?</u> Give example of either or both if applicable.

_____

_____

C. Is employee's <u>initiative</u> expressed in <u>areas not related</u> to <u>immediate job</u> or primarily to <u>job setting</u> and <u>requirements?</u>
Please give examples. _____

_____

_____

VII. ORGANIZING ABILITY (effectiveness in planning and performing work systematically)

A. Is time <u>effectively used</u> in performing tasks? _____

B. How well does employee plan work? Priorities? _____

C. Is employee capable of <u>organizing activities of others</u> in addition to his own? Has this happened?
Please give an example.

_____

_____

VIII. DEVELOPMENT AND TRAINING

A. In order of importance, state performance characteristics which need improvement.

1. _____

2. _____

3. _____

ADDENDUM E *(Cont'd)*

B. What specific steps are you and the employee taking to improve overall job performance? _____

_____

_____

C. Is/Has this employee (been) involved in any formal training or related program outside of work? If so, what is subject matter? How is employee doing?

_____

_____

IX. SUPERVISORY ABILITY

A. How well does employee <u>supervise</u> and/or <u>train</u> <u>staff</u> under direction? _____

_____

B. How might employee be <u>rated</u> overall <u>by</u> his <u>subordinates</u>? <u>Peers</u>? _____

_____

RATING:
☐ Substantially Below Standard
☐ Below Standard
☐ Acceptable
☐ Above Average
☐ Consistently Effective
☐ Exceptional

_____
Employee's Signature

_____
Supervisor's Signature

_____
Department Head or Administrative Signature

EMPLOYEE COMMENTS: _____

_____

_____

_____

_____

_____

_____

_____

ADDENDUM F

THE MOUNT SINAI HOSPITAL

ADMINISTRATIVE APPRAISAL PROGRAM*

Name: _____

Present Position: _____

Date of Hire: _____

CONTENTS

* Excerpt

216

ADDENDUM F *(Cont'd)*

SECTION I — INTRODUCTION

"You cannot teach a man anything. You can only help him to find it within himself," Galileo.

A difficult, yet fundamental step in any well-rounded administrative development program is an objective evaluation of the abilities of the people in the organization. Administrative abilities should be assessed with due regard to the organizational environment in which they are exercised. The difficulty of predicting the capacity of an individual for administrative work has become increasingly important. There is a need for an orderly, objective approach which will enable us to evaluate performance and to inventory the abilities and possible lines of progression for men with potential.

The Mount Sinai Hospital Administrative Appraisal Program aims at reenforcing administrative performance by a systematic assessment of observable work achievements, rather than intangible personality traits. It aims at improvement, not criticism. Emphasis is placed on identifying the individual's capacity through observation of what he actually does rather than what he presumably is.

There is no yardstick that can measure men accurately. The individual factors on the following pages are not of equal weight. In our opinion, however, they are all critical to effective job performance.

The program is divided into three parts:

1. **The Personal Appraisal Form** No. P-134 B, is completed by the administrator whose performance is to be appraised.

   Optimum performance is a mutual goal for the organization and the individual. The primary responsibility for initiating administrative development is left where it belongs—with the individual. Much of the friction which develops in a work situation occurs because there is no clear-cut, mutual agreement about work objectives. This part of the Administrative Appraisal Program gives the individual an opportunity to express his understanding and interpretation of what his job entails, and how well he can meet its requirements.

2. **The Peer Appraisal Form** No. P-134 C, is completed by two colleagues of the administrator (to be selected by the supervisor). Here the individual's performance is appraised by his peers in terms of his contribution to the team effort. Emphasis is on what he does, and whether his performance strengthens or weakens his colleagues' efforts to perform effectively.

3. **The Supervisor Appraisal Form** No. P-134 A, is the part of the Administrative Appraisal Program which should be of most assistance to the supervisor in helping the administrator in his self-development efforts. The supervisor will have the benefit of both the Personal and the Peer Appraisal Forms to assist him in his evaluation.

The factors to be evaluated in the Supervisor Appraisal Form each contain four phrases describing varying degrees of effectiveness. While we fully realize that none of the four phrases may be precisely appropriate, we do request the appraiser to check one of them, for he is given considerable latitude to explain how the phrase is inexact.

SECTION II

PRELIMINARY INSTRUCTIONS

Prior to his appraisal of an administrator's performance, the supervisor must accomplish the following:

(a) **Administrative Appraisal Program Booklet**

Complete the blanks on Page 1 of the Administrative Appraisal Program Booklet by entering the administrator's name, present position and date of hire.

(b) **Personal Appraisal Form**

Complete the blanks on the cover sheet of the Personal Appraisal Form. In addition to the information required in (a) above, this cover sheet should indicate the day, date, time and location set for the Appraisal Interview. The interview should be scheduled to take place 5 or 6 weeks after the date of issue of the Personal Appraisal Form.

The administrator whose performance is being appraised should be allowed three weeks to complete and return the Personal Appraisal Form to the supervisor. The date for return should also be noted on the cover sheet before the form is given to the administrator for completion.

(c) **Peer Appraisal Form**

The two persons who are to complete the Peer Appraisal Forms should be selected on the basis of interrelated responsibilities and close working association with the appraisee-administrator. An administrator's peers are probably best equipped to evaluate his performance realistically. A careful choice is imperative.

Before releasing the Peer Appraisal Form for completion, the supervisor should complete the cover sheets by identifying the appraisee and the peer-appraisers, and by specifying the date that the forms should be returned. Three weeks should be allowed for completion of the Peer Appraisal Forms.

(d) **Supervisor Appraisal Form**

When the Personal Appraisal and Peer Appraisal Forms have been returned to the supervisor, he should study them carefully, for they will aid him in his own evaluation. He should then complete the Supervisor Appraisal Form, and prepare for the Appraisal Interview. (See Section IV)

ADDENDUM F *(Cont'd)*

SECTION III

:UPERVISOR APPRAISAL FORM No. P-134 A
nstructions

1. Review the entire form before you begin the appraisal.
2. Take time to do the job properly. Collect your thoughts, collect your data, e.g., information regarding plans executed, programs started and completed, the administrator's contribution to the Hospital's overall endeavor, etc.
3. Base your assessments on actual performance in the present job. In considering each quality, think over the results obtained.
4. Be on your guard against the common pitfalls in rating:
   (a) Treat each quality separately. Do not allow the administrator's strengths or weaknesses in one quality to affect your appraisal of his other qualities. Avoid a "halo" effect. •
   (b) Do not permit your personal liking for the individual to influence your rating. You are appraising his ability to do the job.
   (c) Avoid the tendency to rate those who hold more important jobs higher than those in less important jobs. Disregard organizational levels when evaluating.
   (d) Some appraisers tend to avoid the extremes of the scale. Avoid this "central" tendency by using very high or very low ratings where the appraisee's performance actually warrants such ratings.
   (e) Be sure that your ratings do not reflect an undue bias toward the extremes of the scale.
5. Rate performance during the past year. The appraisal program is based on the assumption that performance improves with coaching and self-development. This improvement, while slow, should be observable over the course of a year and should be recognized in the appraisal.
6. In each category place an X next to the phrase which most accurately describes the administrator's performance.

PART ONE

A. Professional/Specialist Knowledge

Consider the extent of his professional/specialist knowledge and his ability to apply it in his work situation.

On the basis of his actual performance, indicate which of the following statements is most accurate:

☐ 1. His professional/specialist knowledge enables him to solve most problems satisfactorily;

☐ 2. His professional/specialist knowledge is adequate but he often cannot apply it;

☐ 3. His lack of knowledge frequently makes him unable to cope with technical problems;

☐ 4. Both his professional/specialist knowledge and his ability to apply it are of a high order.

Briefly state instances which have occurred during the past twelve months which illustrate the extent of his professional/specialist knowledge and his ability to apply it. Alternatively, give general comments supporting your rating.

_____
_____
_____
_____
_____
_____
_____
_____
_____

B. Willingness to Assume Responsibility

Consider whether he has shown willingness to take on additional and more responsible duties.

On the basis of his actual performance, indicate which of the following statements is most accurate:

☐ 1. Generally accepts and discharges responsibilities willingly and follows through to conclusion;

☐ 2. Seeks additional responsibility and authority. Carries out projects to satisfactory conclusion;

☐ 3. Unwilling to assume responsibility;

☐ 4. Reluctant to accept responsibility for any but easy projects.

Briefly state instances which have occurred during the past twelve months which illustrate the extent of his willingness to assume responsibility. Alternatively, give general comments supporting your rating.

_____
_____
_____
_____
_____
_____
_____
_____

218

ADDENDUM F *(Cont'd)*

THE APPRAISAL INTERVIEW

At the risk of being redundant, we repeat here that the Administrative Appraisal Program aims, not at criticism, but at improvement of performance through recognition of an administrator's strengths and weaknesses. A sincere acceptance of this philosophy is a primary and essential step in achieving our objective.

The Appraisal Interview should be conducted in complete privacy — including privacy from unexpected visitors, telephone calls or other interruptions. A friendly informal atmosphere should be established. For this purpose, an interview off the Hospital premises might be helpful. It should be made clear to the appraisee that the purpose of the interview is not to criticize, but to reach agreement on plans for improved performance.

There will probably be areas in which the appraiser's evaluation will agree with the administrator's Personal Appraisal. These should be discussed first, and only then should the points of variance be introduced. At all times, the appraisee should be the central figure in the interview. He should be permitted ample opportunity to explain or justify his opinion, and be assured that his reactions are of prime importance. The supervisor should listen and evaluate, recognizing that his own biases and prejudices could have influenced his judgment.

Every interview involves the interaction of two people, each with his own purposes, knowledge, viewpoint and attitudes. While these differences may be difficult to reconcile, a well managed interview can help determine goals and set standards which are mutually acceptable. Both parties may then identify problems which hinder achievement of their goals and arrive at workable solutions. A constructive interview is a valuable management technique which requires the application of considerable skill, thought, and effort.

ADDENDUM F *(Cont'd)*

THE MOUNT SINAI HOSPITAL

ADMINISTRATIVE APPRAISAL PROGRAM

Section V

PERSONAL APPRAISAL FORM No. P-134 B

Name: _____

Present Position: _____

Date of Hire: _____

Supervisory Appraisal Schedule: Day: _____

Date: _____

Time: _____

Location: _____

By: _____

    Optimum performance is a common goal for the Hospital and the individual. In order to strengthen administrative performance, it is essential that a clear-cut mutual agreement be reached as to individual work objectives and plans for their attainment.

    As a key member of the administrative staff, your performance has marked effect upon the successful operation of the hospital. Therefore, within a few weeks, your supervisor will discuss with you his evaluation of your performance over the past year.

    At the time of your appraisal interview, you should be prepared to discuss your job, and what it entails as YOU see it, and to give your own evaluation of your performance. This form has been designed to give you the opportunity to discuss your job in specifics rather than generalities. It is hoped that, thereby, you can be assisted not only to set realistic goals, but to achieve them. Your administrative development is primarily your own responsibility.

To be completed by_____   To be returned to_____
                date

220

ADDENDUM F *(Cont'd)*

HOW WOULD YOU RATE YOUR PERFORMANCE OVER THE PAST YEAR

(Check appropriate point anywhere along scale)

low _____ high

A. Ability to plan for specific goals ....

B. Ability to determine suitable course of action ....

C. Ability to organize for orderly accomplishment ....

D. Ability to motivate others ....

E. Ability to get along with others ....

F. Ability to control people and situations effectively ....

G. Ability to select and train personnel ....

H. Ability to delegate authority and responsibility successfully ....

I. Ability to follow through until required end result is achieved ....

221

ADDENDUM G

THE MOUNT SINAI HOSPITAL
NEW YORK·

PERSONNEL EVALUATION FORM
NURSING PROFESSIONAL PERSONNEL

NAME:	POSITION:
LIFE NO.:	ASSIGNMENT:
SUPERVISOR:	EVALUATED BY:
DATE OF EMPLOYMENT:	TYPE OF EVALUATION:
DATE OF TERMINATION:	☐ Annual ☐ Probationary ☐ Reference ☐ Termination ☐ Promotion

OVERALL EVALUATION (Check appropriate point on scale)

SUPERIOR	ABOVE AVERAGE	AVERAGE (SATISFACTORY)	FAIR	POOR (UNSATISFACTORY)

Explanation:

Superior — Outstanding nurse; sets excellent example to associates and auxiliary personnel; recognized as responsible professional.

Above Average — Maintains high standards, displays initiative.

Average — Performs at satisfactory level, minimum initiative but can be depended upon to follow instructions.

Fair — Seldom displays initiative, performs at minimal level, seldom does more than is required. Needs follow-up.

Poor — Unsatisfactory performance, requires frequent follow-up.

SUMMARY

Give a concise but complete summary of nurse's attitude, personal qualifications, relationship with patients and professional acumen. Please note any points of significance not adequately covered in factor ratings.

PRINCIPLE STRENGTHS: _____

_____

AREAS TO BE IMPROVED: _____

_____

ADDITIONAL COMMENTS: _____

_____

222

I RELATIONSHIP WITH PATIENTS

Evaluate employee's ability to develop rapport with visitors, family, and understand the needs of patient:

0. Little or no interest in patient; often cold and abrupt   0
1. Detached, but not unpleasant   1
2. Displays awareness and sensitivity to patients problems and needs   2
3. Exceptional interest in patient; patient-orientated; engenders good will   3

II RELATIONSHIPS WITH OTHERS

Consider cooperation with peers, success in building and maintaining respect and loyalty of subordinates, and attitude towards supervisor:

0. Displays lack of regard for associates   0
1. Usually cooperative, but not always tactful   1
2. Meets others half-way, is respected by associates   2
3. Engenders good-will, displays and earns loyalty and regard. Consistently builds good relationships   3

III PROFESSIONAL CAPABILITY

Evaluate the employee's application of nursing principles and bedside nursing techniques:

0. Below acceptable standards for present assignment   0
1. Minimum ability, fair technique   1
2. Carries out assignments with care and accuracy   2
3. Superior capability, expert on job   3

IV GROWTH POTENTIAL

Consider participation in professional organizations and interest in furthering education:

0. Will not or cannot accept more responsibility   0
1. Accepts responsibility, shows interest in growth   1
2. Versatile, ambitious; displays ability for increased responsibility   2

V ATTITUDE TOWARDS HOSPITAL

0. Does not reflect understanding and appreciation of Hospital's objectives   0
1. Loyal employee; accepts supervision   1
2. Extremely "Hospital-Oriented" resulting in high morale of associates   2

VI PERSONAL QUALIFICATIONS

Consider appearance, vitality, grooming and personal hygiene:

0. Unkempt, slovenly   0
1. Neat, fit and applies principles of personal hygiene   1
2. Superior appearance and grooming   2

223

DEFINITION OF TRAITS

I. RELATIONSHIP WITH PATIENTS

An important aspect of a nurse's job is her ability to develop rapport and understanding with the patient.
  A. Consider her approach to the patient's well-being.
  B. Consider her attitude towards family and visitors.
  C. Does she display understanding of basic physical, emotional and spiritual needs of patient?
  D. Is she flexible in dealing with the differences in patients due to economic levels, emotional stability, and medical histories?
  E. Does she show a sincere concern for people?
As a nurse who is pleasant to patients, but somewhat detached, should be rated near the middle of the scale.

II. RELATIONSHIP WITH OTHERS

Consider this factor as a measurement of the employee's demonstrated ability to work harmoniously with others.
    The employee who is reasonably pleasant, cooperates when asked, causes no friction but does not increase the spirit of the group, is about average and should be rated near the middle of the scale.
    To be rated at the top of the scale, the employee should be an individual who goes out of her way to cooperate, thus stimulating willingness and cooperation on the part of others.

III. PROFESSIONAL CAPABILITY

We are concerned here with the nurse's performance; her application of nursing principles.
  A. Consider her ability to organize and complete assignments.
  B. Consider the degree of care necessary in carrying out procedures.
  C. Consider care of equipment.
  D. Does she exercise sound judgment in dealing with problems of patients?
  E. Does she display depth of understanding of techniques and details?
The employee who is satisfactory, no more or less than acceptable, should be rated in the middle of the scale.

IV. GROWTH POTENTIAL

We are measuring the nurse's demonstrated ability to accept additional responsibility and diversified assignments.
  A. This factor is also measured in displayed-interest in in-service programs, professional organizations and further education.
An employee who accepts the responsibilities of her assignments, no more or less, should be rated in the middle of the scale.

V. ATTITUDE TOWARDS HOSPITAL

Morale and, in turn, effectivity are greatly affected by the employee's motivation. Closely tied-in with the nurse's motivation is her attitude toward the Hospital.
The nurse who readily accepts supervision, understands and is sympathetic to the administration's goals and purposes should be rated in the middle of the scale.

VI. PERSONAL QUALIFICATIONS

We are concerned here with the nurse's appearance and grooming.
  A. Are her uniforms clean, neat and well-fitted?
  B. Does she maintain good posture?
  C. Does she apply good principles of personal hygiene?
A nurse who is always well-groomed and sets an example for others should be rated near the top of the scale.

VI. TRAINING AND DEVELOPMENT

One of the more important functions of the health care administrator is training. It is important because it gives to the employee and to the administration what each desires without taking away anything from the other. The training of employees can be defined as a process of aiding them to gain effectiveness in the performance of their duties as they are presently understood, or in any future assignment, through the development of appropriate habits of thought, action, skills, knowledge and attitudes. It is through the vehicle of training that attempts are made to communicate skills and attitudes.

There are certain precepts which must be explored and understood before embarking upon any discussion of the training function: [1]

1. Training is an all-permeating function which goes on from day-to-day and cannot be considered an appendage or a necessary evil. It is a ubiquitous process directed toward maximizing employees' efforts in the work arena and culminating in a more effective, cohesive organization.

2. Motivation is an essential part of training—it is important to consider the motivations of both the employees and the administration before developing a training program.

3. Training is a costly but productive undertaking. Although there is a growing skepticism as to the eventual "payoff" of training programs, a careful screening of trainees and careful development of curriculae will ensure such success. No matter how wide or narrow any applied program of training may be, essentially it is a method and a means of communication. Through training we communicate skills, methods, ideas, information, objectives and last, but by no means least, attitudes.

Training in the Health Services Environment

Training is certainly not a new concept nor a new responsibility in the health services industry. The prototype of training in the hospital is the extremely formalized and sophisticated approach toward preparing doctors for general practice and specialization. It is from this model that the nursing departments throughout the health care system have patterned their own in-service training program. For years training was conducted on a de-

225

centralized basis, albeit centralized as to controls within departments. The nursing department maintained in-service training of registered nurses, licensed practical nurses and nurses' aides through the central nursing office. Other specialties in the hospital implemented their own training programs. Although one authority has commented, "Hospitals generally have no great tendency to embrace training programs during recent years,"[2] a trend can now be seen toward centralization of formalized training throughout the hospital industry. Many large health care institutions have delegated the responsibility for developing and overseeing hospital-wide training to training sections within their personnel departments. Bennett predicted, "Looking to the future, I think that with the vast expansion of technology, management systems and computerizations on the one hand, and the increasing financial involvement of the government in caring for the nation's sick and aged on the other, hospitals will be susceptible to increasing activity from non-hospital sources regarding their efficiency. If they are to pass these tests, it will mean among other things that hospitals require more and better equipped people."[3] To accomplish this latter goal, many health care institutions have established highly sophisticated and productive training programs.

Many of these programs were sparked by the statement of the American Hospital Association on the role and responsibility of the hospitals for in-service education: "The hospital in discharging its responsibility for the quality of care rendered to patients has the obligation to assure patients that those who provide service are competent to do so."[4] It was clearly a time of movement from the acceptance of below-standard, marginal workers to an era of higher standards and formalized programs to produce more efficient work forces. Three elements appear to be at the heart of the changeover from ad hoc, fragmented training to centralized and pervasive programs:

1. Wages and fringe benefits reached new levels and the "cheap" labor supply, once so prevalent in health care institutions disappeared. Unionization of health care workers produced higher and more competitive wage scales and broad (even esoteric in some cases) fringe benefit programs.

2. Turnover, always high in health care institutions, was no longer acceptable based upon the salary level of health care workers and the obvious inefficiency inherent in short-term employment.

3. The cost of recruitment, now more discernible through highly sophisticated record-keeping, was intolerable. Most studies indicate that the replacement cost at the lowest level of skill is approximately $300, while many health care workers fall into semiskilled, skilled and professional categories where the cost runs more nearly to $1,000 per employee.

Commencing in 1960, health care institutions began to recognize that it was good business to establish formalized training programs for some or all of the following reasons:

1. The break in time for new employees can be sharply decreased.

2. Efficiency levels, once recognized, can be attained through appropriate training.

3. Waste, spoilage, accidents—all can be reduced by properly trained employees.

4. Research has clearly indicated that employee dissatisfaction expressed in absenteeism, tardiness and turnover often is a product of ill-trained and ill-equipped employees. Training programs, therefore, can measurably reduce such personnel problems.

5. Employees can be prepared for higher positions and more responsibilities through intensive training. Those to be considered for supervisory positions, once chosen on an ad hoc basis and on less than scientific criteria, can now be identified (assessment centers) and trained (management development).

6. Training can improve job satisfaction and morale and reduce grievances.

The intensification of third-party review of hospital finances magnified the need for more efficient labor forces. Labor was no longer the cheap commodity it had been. This fact and the federal government's heightened interest in health care during the 1960's combined to produce an incentive toward improved training programs in health care institutions. The federal government sponsored training of health care personnel through the Manpower Development and Training Act of 1962. In 1963 the Health Professions Assistant Act was passed. In 1964 the Nurse Training Act; in 1966, the Allied Health Professions Personnel Training Act; and in 1970, the Health Training Improvement Act. This latter act (P.L. 91-519) extends the Allied Health Professions Act. It broadens the special projects and traineeships section by making funds available to private agencies, organizations and institutions as well as training centers for allied health professions. Section 202 of the act authorized $45 million over three years, 1971 through 1973, to assist training centers in developing new or improved curriculae for training allied health professions personnel; otherwise, to improve the quality of their educational programs. Section 203 authorized $30 million over the same three years to cover cost of traineeships of personnel to teach health service technicians or any of the allied health professions specialties determined by the Surgeon General to require advanced training. In addition to governmental assistance for training in the health care field, the

W. K. Kellogg Foundation has funded many diversified health education projects.

Still another source of impetus to improve training developed through the advent of collective bargaining agreements. In the agreement between the State of New York and the Civil Service Employees Association (Institution Services Unit, 1972-1973), one finds the following article:

> There shall be training programs designed to develop knowledge and skills of employees. Specific training programs may provide remedial training, lead to high school equivalency diplomas or develop skills for improved on-the-job performance and advancement through career ladders and otherwise . . . . The State will recommend an appropriation by the legislature of $1 million for the fiscal year 1972-73 for implementation of such training programs.

In the agreement between the League of Voluntary Hospitals and Homes of New York City and Local 1199, the Drug and Hospital Union, RWDSU, AFL-CIO, covering over 40 hospitals and homes, one finds this clause:

> The parties shall continue planning for and training adequate health personnel for institutions covered by this agreement through the Hospital League-Local 1199 Training and Upgrading Fund. The Hospitals shall pay to the trustees of such fund an amount equal to one percent (1%) of the gross payroll of employees exclusive of employees who have not completed two months of employment. Contributions so received by the trustees shall be used to study hospital manpower needs including shortages and entry level jobs, upgraded positions and credential jobs; to develop career ladders and subsidize employees in training and when necessary, the cost of training in areas of manpower shortages. Such programs shall be administered under an agreement and declaration of trust. Trustees of such training and upgrading funds, in addition to the monies received from hospitals, shall attempt to secure such additional funds as may be available from public or other private sources. In addition, the trustees shall seek community cooperation in such programs.

The federal government, private foundations, collective bargaining agreements and third-party intervention in the financial viability of such institutions directed the attention of hospital administrators to an area once thought of as too expensive, too time-consuming and too unimportant.

Training Objectives and Truths

It has been stated that there are three basic objectives of any training program.

1. The acquisition of knowledge.
2. The development of skill.
3. The development or modification of attitudes. Stokes warns that the person responsible for employee training must be constantly on guard and aware of the problems inherent in this responsibility:[5]

1. Training takes time. It is often in competition with the other activities (the central activities of the institution). Since it is time consuming, successful results must be highlighted for those sponsoring a training program.

2. Training costs money. The trainee who becomes a highly skilled and productive worker must be considered worthy of a rather high hourly investment.

3. Employers want to retain trained help. One of the often heard protestations against training programs is that "We don't want to train people for other institutions." With a little extra effort and attention, it is possible to retain trained people, especially when area wage rates are quite similar and there is not much wage advantage in moving from one institution to another.

4. Small institutions especially need training. Although larger institutions can have complete training departments that recruit trainees, set up professional programs, retain topnotch trainers and spread the training course over a large budget, smaller institutions are limited in such matters. Once it is determined that training is necessary, regardless of the size of the institution, it is possible to run a successful program.

5. Training requires administrative time. Training is not an activity that can be isolated from other functions of the institution. Even though administration has assigned the conduct of a program to certain specialists, it must constantly support training, be aware of the results obtained and be certain training is properly and effectively carried out.

6. Training must be done by specialists. The person who does the training must be chosen because of his technical skill and knowledge. Every technically competent supervisor must become an effective developer of people. It is one of his prime responsibilities to train his own help.

Before embarking upon a total training program, one must try to discern all the problems—those previously listed and those (even more obvious) not listed. The resistance to training is not limited to the top administrative cadre. First-line administrators are often more forceful and vehement in their resistance to the time and cost of training. It is not unusual to hear such supervisors complain about released time and the lack of immediate results from training. Often when the training is a vestibule program, given in advance of the new employee's assignment to the department, the supervisor will press for immediate release of the new employee to the work area. It is therefore the responsibility of the personnel administrator to carefully plan the training program and sell it to all levels of the administration (see Exhibit 1). If training is truly the process of assisting employees toward becoming more effective in their present or future assignments within the institution, then with a sensitive presentation to the administration the personnel administrator can overcome the problems of natural resistance to such efforts. It is well to remember and to "market" the following truism: "Training aims to increase the effectiveness with which the functions of an organization are carried out through increasing the effectiveness of the personnel comprising that organization."[6]

Policy on Training

The goals of the training program must be clearly defined and communicated. This may be accomplished by establishing a policy on training adopted by the board of trustees and underwritten by the chief administrative officer of the institution. The policy must indicate how training will be carried out, who will be responsible for its administration, the types involved in the overall program, the relationship of line to staff in the implementation and how the costs will be borne. It must also indicate how employees will be paid for the time spent in institutionally directed training. Training conducted during regular working hours offers no difficulty. The employee is paid his regular salary for such participation. If the scheduled sessions fall outside the employee's work area, it is not unusual to give the employee either pay for such hours or a compensatory day off during the same pay period. Another important element of the training policy is the selection of trainees. Since more emphasis is being placed on selection of employees who are exposed to training, careful review of qualifications, abilities and, in many cases, testing of potential trainees may well be part of the selection process. The "how" of such selection should be clearly delineated. If there are seniority requirements, often present in unionized situations, these should be communicated in the policy statement.

Planning the Training Program

Odiorne suggests four rules which might prevent a failure in training:[7]
1. Establish the training need through some evidence.
2. Devise the training program around these needs.
3. Execute it in a professional manner.
4. Evaluate its effectiveness.

A detailed discussion of the first two points is necessary before exploration of the latter two. Training needs can be established through the following evidence:

Exhibit 1
Suggested Outline for Proposal for Training Program or Activity*

[date]

TO: [*administrative officer*]

FROM: [*training director*]

SUBJECT: Proposal for [*title of program or activity*]

I. We [*identify persons involved*] have found the following learning needs:
   [*specify A or B*]:
   A. Immediate learning needs related to [*identify performance deficiencies*] on the part of
      [*identify by job classification and department*]
   B. Long-range learning needs related to [*identify performance deficiencies*] on the part of
      [*identify by job classification and department*] ·

II. These needs were made evident by [*indicate relevant items from the following*]:
   A. Changes in [*specify service, equipment, procedures, staffing patterns*]
   B. Employee records of [*work performance, turnover, absenteeism*]
   C. Reports of [*incidents, accidents, equipment and supply usage, patient complaints*]
   D. Interviews with [*department heads, supervisors, and/or employees*]
   E. On-the-job observations of [*work performance, work flow, procedures*]
   F. Questionnaire survey(s) of [*specify employee groups*]
   G. Requests from employees for [*specify programs or activities requested*]

III. To meet these needs we recommend a program(s) with the following objectives [*specify
   learning objectives, in performance terms whenever possible*]:

IV. To meet the stated objectives, the program(s) will be developed for the following personnel
   [*list by name, by department, or by classification*]:

V. Tentative outline of proposed program(s):
   A. Time schedule [*dates and hours*]
   B. Major topics and/or activities [*specify*]
   C. Methods of instruction to be used [*specify*]
   D. Instructors

VI. Estimated budget [*dollars or man-hours — relevant items from the following*]:
   A. Time of employees [*if during working hours, estimate class hours per person*]
   B. Time of instructors, coordinator, and/or meeting leaders
   C. Cost of facilities and materials [*classroom space or outside facility rental, audiovisual
      media, handouts, reference materials, etc.*]
   D. Honoraria for guest speakers
   E. Other [*reimbursed travel expenses, meals or refreshments for participants and guest
      speakers, etc.*]

VII. The program(s) will be evaluated as follows [*specify*]:

**Training and Continuing Education: A Handbook for Health Care Institutions* (Chicago: Hospital
Research & Education Trust, 1970), p. 4.

1. Manpower shortage or inadequate supplies of employees who are promotable.

2. Specific skill shortages within the institution and/or in the labor market in general.

3. General employee dissatisfaction as expressed in large numbers of grievances, excessive turnover and unacceptable levels of disciplinary problems.

4. Patient complaints about service.

5. Inability of departments to function within proscribed budgetary restraints.

6. Poor morale level.

7. Union activity, either expressed in new drives toward collective employee action or in increased drives in already organized institutions.

8. Development of new policies or contractual agreements which must be communicated, understood and implemented by administrative and supervisory groups.

9. Ineffective supervisory techniques.

Without the accumulation of factual evidence of need, little can be expected from training programs. Programs must be developed on the basis of information, which should indicate the desired areas of concentration. A reliable roster of actual skills must be assembled and a differentiation made between potential skills and actual skills. These skill inventories often may be included as a part of the computer base on employees. They are of immeasurable assistance in determining promotable individuals and highlighting areas of training concentration. Surveys of supervisors *on available skills and projected needs* over the next several years should be an integral part of planning for the training of present and future employees. In addition to establishing the skill scarcities, those individuals within the organization who need training must be identified. Still another part of the training rubric is the establishment of the types of training that will be included in the general plan. Some of these approaches include:

1. On-the-job training.
2. Conferences.
3. Lectures.
4. Role-playing.
5. Sensitivity training.
6. Assessment centers.

On-the-Job Training

Most training is done by supervisors and senior employees. This type of one-to-one training is conducted on the job and often informally. There is a perceptible tendency toward training of individuals rather than groups. An increasing proportion of all training done in health care institutions is conducted by supervisors or fellow workers rather than by members of a formal training department. The most successful approach to on-the-job training is the four-step method of instruction.

1. *Preparing the trainer: setting an atmosphere of receptivity.* This is the most critical phase of the teaching job. Its main thrust is to establish a *mood* and general *attitude* in the trainee which will produce a willingness to accept the training which follows. Successful trainers spend more time preparing to train than in actual training. In order to properly facilitate this section of the basic training pattern, the trainer should have carefully reviewed the trainee's background. Prior training exposure should be ascertained. It is during this first step that the trainee's interest should be aroused. Key suggestions for the successful implementation of this step include establishing an atmosphere of informality; introduction of both the trainee and the trainer; personal review of past work assignments to establish a base of departure; determining the importance of the job and how the trainee will benefit by being exposed to the training program.

This latter point deserves careful attention. It is the "what's in it for me" syndrome too often underrated by so-called sophisticated trainers. The effectiveness of communicating the worth of the training in the short run and long run of the employee's career often has a direct effect on how quickly he will learn and, in some cases, if he will learn at all. If training is to be successful, it should be a challenge to the trainee; it should be something the trainee really wants to do; it should be tied into the trainee's overall career aspirations; and it should be within the normal grasp of the trainee as far as understanding and ability to absorb the material.

In review, this first step directs its attention to putting the trainee at ease and getting him personally involved and interested in the job, thus establishing a desire to learn.

2. *Demonstrating the parts of the job: tell and show.* Much of what one learns is the result of seeing. A lesser amount results from being told. The most effective training, therefore, results from telling and showing. In demonstrating the job, it is most important to plan the presentation in advance. This includes establishing a job breakdown sheet (see Exhibit 2, page 234). This sheet establishes the important steps in the operation. A step is defined as a logical segment of the operation when something happens to advance the work. Alongside each of these steps, key points are outlined. A key point is anything in a step that might *make or break* the job or make the work easier to do. The trainer may forget the why and pass over key points which he, himself, takes for granted. A job breakdown sheet can minimize such prob-

LIBRARY ST. MARY'S COLLEGE

Exhibit 2

Job Break-Down Sheet for Training Man on New Job

Operation. . . . .

IMPORTANT STEPS IN THE OPERATION	KEY POINTS
Step: A logical segment of the operation when something happens to ADVANCE the work.	Key Point: Anything in a step that might: Make or break the job, Injure the worker, Make the work easier to do, i.e., "knack," "trick," special timing, bit of special information.
1.) Take carton from rack.	Keep 4-section cover flaps well bent back.
2.) Grasp six boxes at a time from drop feed.	
3.) Place boxes in carton and repeat until filled.	
4.) Insert instruction sheet.	
5.) Insert excelsior packing. Close 4-section cover flaps.	Grasp instruction sheet and excelsior at the same time. It saves time and makes sure both are inserted.
6.) Remove full carton from table.	Slide, do not lift full cartons onto removing chute. This preserves strength and prevents accidents.

lems. Too often the trainer instructs in the order in which the job is performed, whereas it may be a great deal easier to break the job down into different segments (not necessarily in order) since some of the steps may be quite easy for the individual to learn while others may be difficult. In demonstrating, it is best to proceed from the known to the unknown: teach the simple first and lead up to the complicated. Too often the trainer thinks of the job in much larger units than can be absorbed by the trainee. Attention must be directed to the need for the steps to be digestible. It is important to explain each step as it is being demonstrated and to explain why that particular approach is taken.

Tell and Show incorporates a willingness on the part of the trainer to answer questions. Therefore, the trainee should be encouraged (by establishing that initial permissive atmosphere) to ask questions at any point in the demonstration.

3. *Performance by the trainee.* This is the first opportunity for the trainee to do the actual job himself. It can be done after all the job's parts are demonstrated or after a single part or a combination of several parts is demonstrated. The trainee should be required to explain what he will be doing before he does it. Do not permit the trainee to *learn in error.* If in his explanation he appears to be embarking upon an improper approach to the job, he should be stopped, reinstructed on the procedure and then permitted to perform. When he performs, he should outline the key points. After successfully performing the job, he should be permitted to continue without interruption unless errors are obvious. Learning by repetition is a most important element of on-the-job training. As the trainee performs more efficiently, less and less time is needed in supervision.

4. *Follow-up and review.* A formal program should be developed to check on the trainee's progress. The trainer should return at intervals to establish the effectiveness of the training. He must determine what additional training is needed to reinforce the trainee. The trainee should always be encouraged to call for help. Coaching is an integral part of this step and should be available as needed.

A modification of on-the-job training is the vestibule approach to instruction of employees. This self-contained vestibule training center is separated from the actual work area and simulates actual on-the-job working conditions. It offers the advantage of less pressure and remedies a most prevalent disadvantage to normal on-the-job training: the supervisor's impatience with trainees based upon day-to-day needs in the work area. On-the-job training is often ineffective because of the pressures and needs of the daily operation. The vestibule approach minimizes such pressures.

Conferences

Without a doubt the most widely used method of training in health care institutions is the conferences. This method offers the participants the unusual opportunity to contribute ideas, exchange experiences and solve problems by means of *pooled judgment.* Through peer pressure, participants often rethink previously untouchable positions within the context of the group. The essence of the conference is the drawing together of employees with varying skills, experiences and responsibilities in order for group members to learn from each other, rather than from a trainer. The success of the conference is largely dependent upon its composition and the skill of the conference leader.

Who Shall Attend?

There are two basic methods in grouping employees at conferences. In one instance the group may be a homogeneous one. The participants come from the same area of operations in the institution, but are at different levels of responsibility. For example, a conference of this composition (vertical grouping) in the nursing department envisions participants at the head nurse level, supervisor level and assistant director of nursing level. All group members are familiar with the operation of their department since they are all members of the same department. A second method may offer a hetero-geneous grouping (horizontal method). Here, although all the participants are in a similar level of authority in the organization, they come from different disciplines. A department head conference under this latter method would include the head of food service, the head of building service, the director of nursing, etc. The advantages of this horizontal grouping method over the vertical are the opportunities to exchange ideas from various vantage points in the institution and the absence of restraint in-herent in a grouping that brings together superiors and subordinates as in the vertical method.

Another key consideration is the size of the group. Too large a group (in excess of 20) does not afford all members maximum opportunity to par-ticipate. Very often within the setting of a large conference, small numbers of participants dominate the group. The ideal number is somewhere be-tween 12 and 15, although a skilled conference leader can deal with larger numbers. Still another consideration is the time and setting of the meeting. In the health care institution, pressures are diffuse and the order of the day too often is crisis-oriented. Careful selection of dates, times and places of conferences is necessary to minimize apprehension and interruption. Al-though it may at times be frustrating and, indeed, difficult to arrive at a consensus, it is advisable to survey the members of the group to establish the best day of the week, the best time of the day and the best place for the conference to be held.

The Conference Leader

The ideal conference leader knows the topic, has planned the conference completely and is fully aware of its goals. It is his responsibility to introduce the topic and to motivate the participants to obtain maximum input. He must keep the discussion moving and yet, to be effective, must be unobtrusive. His key roles are to keep the group on the track, summarize any conclusions which develop and, of course, strive to reach the goal(s) of the conference. The experienced conference leader must be able to deal with the overactive conferee who dominates the conference. Conversely, he must encourage the timid participants in order to obtain balanced contributions from the group. Black and Ford suggest a check list for effective conference management:[8]

1. Make certain the subject is worth a meeting.
2. Plan carefully.
3. Work out a plan of action.
4. Inspect the meeting room.
5. Know the participants.
6. Review your responsibilities.
7. Don't forget follow-up.

Too often conferences are called to discuss matters which can be handled in a more expeditious manner. Remember, time is valuable and conferences for conference sake only are wasteful. Planning the agenda is essential in the success of the conference and a timetable is most helpful. In working out the plan of action, it is important to minimize time-consuming activities and to assemble and provide facts to establish a sound frame of reference for the conference. The meeting room should be large enough to hold the group, well-ventilated and with appropriate training aids such as blackboards, charts and pads. A U-shaped table is best suited for most conferences. The conference leader must (to get the meeting off to a good start) initially define the problem(s) precisely and clearly. He should be directing the conference to a consensus and should know the appropriate time to end the meeting. The follow-up procedure includes distribution of any summary of findings and careful attention to "for action" matters.

Lectures

Where time is a factor and large numbers of trainees are involved, the lecture is often the preferred vehicle for disseminating information and communicating new methods and policies. This is basically a "telling" method. The trainer or lecturer presents material in an authoritative manner. Interruptions are limited and participation, unfortunately, is minimized. Often the lecture is an integral part of other methods such as the conference, role-playing or even sensitivity training. By presenting facts in this fashion the trainee or listener has time to digest these facts and draw his own conclusions after the session. Although this method requires less preparation than any other method, there are some key considerations in maximizing the effect of lectures:

1. Set the goals and desired action in advance of the lecture. Keep them constantly in thr forefront, build gradually toward full exploration of the problem and direct the audience's attention to the goals.

2. Understand the group and consider the audience's needs. This is a most difficult aspect of the presentation since many groups are heterogeneous in make-up.

3. Although notes are extremely important, actual reading of them should be limited. Move around as much as possible without affecting the ability of the audience to hear your presentation.

4. Opening remarks should be carefully planned to maximize listeners' interest and arouse listeners' receptivity.

5. Use visual aids where possible. Intersperse reading of material with direct eye focus on parts of the audience and make use of selected visual aids. In using such visual aids, limit the time the speaker's back is to the audience.

6. Prevent boredom by varying the tone and method of presentation; use handouts, blackboard and, where possible, participants.

The chief disadvantage of the lecture is that trainee participation is minimized, and therefore maintaining interest is difficult. This can be overcome by using more than one speaker, i.e., a panel of speakers. In addition, question-and-answer periods help to bridge the gap between the one-way communication of the lecture and the needed two-way exchange for effecting change.

Role-Playing

> If you really understand another person . . . enter his private world
> and see how living appears to him . . . you run the risk of being changed
> yourself. You might see it his way; you might find yourself influenced in
> your attitude or personality.[9]

Role-playing is a very useful technique in developing skills and can be incorporated along with other methods such as conferences, sensitivity training and transactional analysis, and as part of didactic presentations. It may be used in teaching any kind of skill training, especially where human relationships are involved. Using this method, an individual can put himself in another person's shoes to see how that person feels, to experiment with new ways of behaving and to understand other people's behavior. Case material can be tailored to the needs and interests of a particular group. In fact, role-playing situations are best developed from material emanating from the group itself. This is a practical exercise, free from theoretical and academic restraints. The great advantage of role-playing is practice in a reality situation where the participants risk making mistakes and learn therefrom. Since it is, indeed, "playing," you can minimize the risks and still retain all other aspects of a real-life dramatic situation. The individuals are able to diagnose the problems of the players and suggest various approaches without necessitating a defensive attitude on the part of the role-takers. *The group teaches and helps itself.* It often is the one method which provides total participation of the group in discussions concerning the subject at hand.

The first step is to get the group to suggest common problems. This usually evolves from a conference or series of conferences. The situation once developed can motivate the group to attempt approaches. The "skit" is then developed. It is best to obtain volunteers to play the various roles. Certain techniques are most useful in role-playing situations: role reversal, doubling, coaching and role rotation. In *role reversal* one individual is left in a role until at a critical time he is asked to change places with the other role-taker. He is then queried about his feelings in his new role. Roles may then be reversed for a second time. This provides each individual with an opportunity to develop insights into both sides of a problem. *Doubling* provides a third player who expresses his feelings and interprets what he thinks each of the players may be thinking. Conversation may develop between the player and the double. Often the double attempts to challenge the player's perception of a situation. *Coaching* is done by the group. The players once acting out a situation are coached by the group to try different methods. This is a most effective approach. *Role rotation* permits everyone in the group to rotate through each position.

Sensitivity Training

Sensitivity laboratories or T (training) or D (development) groups are designed to make participants more aware of the covert factors—the hidden agenda—that can advance or retard a group as it seeks to accomplish its tasks. Such a group is designed to help individuals become more sensitive to the dynamics of working groups. The primary objective is to make participants more aware of their influence on others and aware for the first time of ways in which they may be unconsciously interfering with the work they are consciously trying to do. It is based upon the premise that leadership behavior of a supervisor can seriously hamper his own effectiveness in getting work accomplished through others. His very behavior and his attitudes may be self-defeating without his awareness of why this is so. The sensitivity group is designed to make him aware of why and how he interacts with group members. This method does not rely primarily upon intellectual learning. In fact, didactic methods are usually not a part of the T group. By experiencing frustrations and facing difficulties, by overcoming group problems, participants learn about group dynamics. Sensitivity training is based on the following premises:

1. The essential sources of personal growth and development lie within the participants themselves; no attempt is made to tell them to change or how to change. The participants are helped to see themselves more objectively; then, as they become dissatisfied with certain aspects of their attitudes or behavior, the decision to change or the direction of change is up to them. In this respect, the function of the trainer is primarily to help create the learning conditions under which the trainees can gain new perspectives of themselves and to help the individual trainee as guidance is sought.

2. People in general want control of their own destinies—they want to engage in healthy interpersonal relations with minimum fears and doubts, free from attitudes, feelings and ideas that keep them from being creative, productive and comfortable within themselves and with others.

3. Interaction with other people is necessary for this kind of productive learning. Each person creates for himself as well as for others of his training group a set of mirrors in which values, attitudes and behaviors can be reflected. Free and open communications are encouraged and the trainees are urged to comment openly on what they see and hear and on how they feel.

4. The setting of a climate for learning is essentially a matter of bringing about certain group conditions which permit the individual to learn. These conditions permit interpersonal exposure of ideas and feelings, valid feedback to the individual as to the adequacy of his ideas and feelings, a supportive atmosphere which allows the individual to look at his own inadequacies and an exploratory behavior directed toward testing of new ideas, attitudes and feelings.

5. Finally, personal growth is best promoted in a learning situation in which the individual is respected and his right to be different protected. Sensitivity training encourages an individual to be himself so that he can test his effectiveness in varying situations that make demands upon his leadership skills.[10]

Argyris, one of the foremost exponents of laboratory education, believes that the most effective development in an individual (or an organization) tends to occur as he becomes more aware of himself and therefore accepts himself more. He believes that sensitivity training in a laboratory education program should provide as many opportunities as possible for the executives to:

1. *Expose their behavior* as well as their thinking.

2. *Receive feedback* about their behavior and give feedback about the behavior of others.

3. *Create an atmosphere* where human beings are willing to expose their values, attitudes and feelings and where they are able to give or receive effective feedback.

4. *Intellectualize the learning* into a rational, consistent, cognitive framework.

5. *Experiment with new ideas, values and behavior.*[11]

One of the criticisms of sensitivity groups comes from psychiatrists who compare such exposure to group therapy and suggest the need for a very careful screening of participants and a careful review of the credentials of the T-group organizer and leader. Very often a highly defensive individual will find this experience most disturbing. It is the relatively healthy individual capable of learning who should be selected for such an experience. Back questions the gain from exposure to T groups for people who feel that they have been "pushed" into such a training experience: "Indiscriminate exposure of these persons to stresses of intensive interpersonal experiences, which they have not sought, is morally hard to justify. It may also have dangerous effects."[12] It would appear that the success of sensitivity training in an institution is greatly dependent upon the careful selection of the participants and the commitment of the participants' superiors to permit the trying out of new ideas and styles developed from such exposure.

Assessment Centers

The origin of the use of multiple assessment procedures on a large scale is credited to the German military psychologists. The British adapted the procedures to the screening of officer candidates, and the United States Office of Strategic Services took over the approach from the British during World War II. Since that time several studies of various applications of these procedures have been reported. Many of the procedures employed have involved multiple methods for obtaining information on individuals, standardization of methods and inferential procedures. In addition, it is quite common to find the use of several assessors whose judgments are polled in arriving at evaluations of the persons assessed.

A major contribution of the multiple assessment approach has been the use of situational tests or exercises. Though not restricted to multiple assessment, the application of situational techniques to assessment has been featured in such programs as that of the OSS. Situational methods offer the potential of adding greatly to the scope of human characteristics which can be evaluated. Though more expensive and time-consuming to administer than other appraisal procedures, the need to find ways of evaluating characteristics not covered by the latter is sufficient to warrant extensive experimentation with relatively elaborate techniques.

Assessment procedures also contrast with psychometric ones in the way the resulting data are combined. Psychometric approaches depend on mathematical methods for accomplishing this purpose, whereas assessment approaches combine the data judiciously. At the present time at least 11 major companies are known to make extensive use of the assessment center approach. Some government agencies also have such programs. Assessment centers are more effective than the usual appraisal procedures because all assessees (1) have an equal opportunity to display their talents, (2) are seen under similar conditions and situations designed to bring out the particular skills and abilities needed for the position or positions for which they are being considered, and (3) are evaluated by a team of trained assessors unbiased by past association who are intimately familiar with the position requirements. By far the largest application of the assessment approach is in selecting applicants for management positions. In these situations the institution is primarily interested in estimating management potential, but centers may also produce training and development recommendations. Although this topic could well be discussed under recruitment or evaluation, it is included in this chapter since it has been effectively used in developing a continuing pool of competent administrators. More and more organizations are designing systematic manpower planning programs including formal management assessment centers to identify and develop tomorrow's managers today.[13]

Presently there is no formal method of assessing the potential of health services personnel candidates before they are promoted or transferred into managerial positions. Before designing a management assessment program for a health care institution, there are several considerations that should be kept in mind. The proposed program should meet as a minimum the following specifications:

1. It must *validly* measure management potential. Decisions made on the potential and development of the individual must be related to actual job performance factors.

2. It must have high *face validity* or acceptability to both the health care institution and the persons being assessed.

3. It must be administered as an integral part of the health care institution's manpower development program. The assessment program should serve as a partial individual needs analysis since the output reports will include information about the individual's skills which may be improved through education, development or training programs. Further, the program should serve as a developmental experience for the assessors (line supervisors) who should have an opportunity to enhance their skills in evaluating performance.

4. It must be *flexible* enough to permit assessment of management potential at various levels and functional areas of specialization and provide for future alterations if the need arises.

5. It must be *comprehensive* enough to tap a wide variety of managerial potential characteristics. The complexity and breadth of managerial functions require an elaborate battery of measuring devices for adequate coverage.

6. It must have a *high payoff value* in relation to investment and cost of administration.

7. It must be *feasible* in terms of the realities of the institution's particular organizational structure and climate, as well as *practically* and theoretically sound.

The assessment center method includes psychological testing with the use of a battery of tests including those for mental ability, numerical ability, logical thinking and personality. A systematical, patterned interview usually follows consisting of a reservoir of preplanned questions to be asked of all candidates. The interviewer evaluates the participant on the basis of his actions and words in the interview. This is usually followed by an "in-basket" exercise. A case history is developed and the participant is asked to put himself in the role of an administrator in that situation. He will then make judgments, delegate assignments and indicate decisions.

The "in-basket" exercise is followed by a leaderless group discussion. This is a semi-structured exercise designed to measure a number of variables that together make up a large part of what is called leadership ability. This exercise requires that the assessees be seated around a table. Observers are in attendance but, of course, do not participate. The group is briefed on the assigned topic for discussion or a problem is posed to the group for solution. The group then is left to its own devices. Each observer takes notes on an assigned number of participants. The variables to be assessed by the observers are leadership, interpersonal relations, flexibility, oral skills and quality of participation. See the Addendum to this chapter for further discussion of an assessment program used at a large voluntary hospital.[14]

Supervisory Training

The job of a supervisor has become increasingly complex in the industrial world. It is far more complex in the health care industry. Supervisory training or management development is "an individual process involving the interaction of a man, his job, his manager and the total work environment . . . (which) results in the acquisition of new knowledge, skills and attitudes in a planned, orderly manner to improve present job performance while accelerating preparation for advancement into more responsible positions."[15] The Conference Board conducted a study of supervisory training programs in 228 firms in the United States and Canada. The responding organizations were engaged in diverse fields of business and varied from small to giant organizations. The findings were most illuminating and have a great deal of relevance to the health care field. Table 1 indicates problems facing first-line supervisors and the organization's responses to them.[16] It is interesting to note that a large majority (160) of the respondents established special training programs for their supervisors whose jobs are changing.

Table 1

Problems Facing First-line Supervisors*

Type of Problem	Number of Responses
Introduction of new methods, technologies, or equipment	124
Poor job attitudes of younger workers	113
Lack of skills of younger workers	107
Lack of skills of disadvantaged workers	88
Poor job attitudes of disadvantaged workers	80
Relationships with employees' union or its agents	75

. . . and the Organization's Response

Establish special training programs, for foremen, apprentices, new workers, workers whose jobs are changing	160
Discuss problems at regularly scheduled supervisory conferences	17
Discuss problems at special supervisory conferences	14
Provide individual counseling by immediate superiors or personnel department, work more closely with supervisors	40
Plan further ahead for the introduction of new methods, change working processes, eliminate paperwork	9
Review, and in some cases change, policies, procedures, employee benefits	9

*Walter S. Wikstrom, *Supervisory Training,* New York: The Conference Board, Inc., 1943, pp. 1-16.

Table 2 reports subjects covered in initial off-the-job training programs in supervisory development. "Leadership," "Leadership skills," "Working with people" or "Human relations" training are the subjects cited most frequently (128 organizations) as part of these training programs.[17] It is obvious that priority consideration in such courses is in the areas of leadership, motivation and management concepts, but many of the programs gave strong emphasis to specific practices of the institutions.

Table 2

Subjects Covered in Initial Off-the-job Training Programs*

Subject Area	Number of Times Mentioned
Leadership, human relations, working with people, behavioral science concepts, motivating employees	128
Management theory and practice, management concepts, the management process	62
Company policies, benefits, personnel procedures	47
Labor relations, labor laws and regulations, collective bargaining, union contracts, dealing with the union	42
Company organization, role of the line departments, role of the staff, staff services	41
Problem solving, analyzing problems, decision making	41
Role of the supervisor, supervisory concepts	30
Safety, firefighting, first aid, housekeeping, the Occupational Safety and Health Act	28
Company administrative procedures, "mechanics," paperwork	27
Company nondiscrimination policy, Equal Employment Opportunity regulations, the minority employee, dealing with minorities	25
Goal-setting, management by objectives	10
Work simplification	10
Economics, the American business system, free enterprise system	6

*Wikstrom, *Ibid.*

Table 3 indicates training methods used for initial off-the-job training and extent used.[18] Group discussion is the most commonly used method and the lecture is the next most frequently used.

Table 4 indicates the types of personnel used as faculty for initial off-the-job training and extent used.[19] Seventy-five percent of the respondents who conduct initial supervisory training courses use training personnel as faculty.

Evaluating Training Results

Although a difficult procedure, it is necessary to institute evaluation methods to ascertain the success or lack of success of specific training and

Table 3

Training Methods Used for Initial Off-the-job Training and Extent Used*

Teaching Method	Number of Respondents	Number of Respondents Reporting Various Percentages of Program Time Devoted to a Given Method				
		0% to 20%	21% to 40%	41% to 60%	61% to 80%	81% to 100%
Group discussion	141	36	69	32	4	
Lecture	137	74	35	23	4	1
Case study	124	100	22	2		
Role playing	106	99	6	1		
Required reading	82	76	5	1		
Business games	51	48	3			
Programmed instruction	38	35	1	2		
Laboratory training	18	15	2	1		

*Wikstrom, *Ibid*.

Table 4

Personnel Used as Faculty for Initial Off-the-job Training and Extent Used*

Faculty Personnel	Number of Respondents	Number of Respondents Reporting Various Percentages of Program Time for Different Faculty Personnel				
		0% to 20%	21% to 40%	41% to 60%	61% to 80%	81% to 100%
Specialized trainers	112	17	11	20	11	53
Other staff personnel	86	45	22	6	4	9
Higher line managers	56	33	5	9	5	4
Present supervisors	25	14	2	4	2	3
Consultants, professors	13	4	2	4		3
Participants themselves	1					1

*Wikstrom, *Ibid*.

development activities. The key question to be answered in this procedure is simply: Is the investment producing the expected results? A subsidiary question is whether the money expended in training endeavors is justified:

> Evaluation is not just a single act or event, but an entire process. It is an intrinsic part of the interrelated activity of determining needs, establishing learning objectives, conducting the program and measuring results.[20]

There is no doubt that most individuals involved in training endeavors in a health care institution are strongly tempted to by-pass the evaluation process. This temptation is born of the fear that the program will appear to be unsupported by its results. The evaluation of training programs is the responsibility of the personnel administrator. He must be familiar with the principles of evaluation:[21]

1. Evaluation.must be conducted in terms of purposes. Each program must be developed with specific goals in order for a determination to be made on its effectiveness. The purposes of the evaluation program must be crystal-clear to all concerned.

2. Evaluation must be cooperative. All who are part of the process of appraisal and all who are affected by it—trainers, trainees, supervisors—must participate in the process.

3. Evaluation must be continuous. It must be a process that never stops, although its form, focus and emphasis may shift.

4. Evaluation must be specific. It must determine what is being done well and what might be done better and how improvements can be made. Specificity is the key.

5. Evaluation must provide the means and focus for trainers to be able to appraise themselves, their practices and their products. The most convincing evaluator is the trainer himself.

6. Evaluation must be based on uniform and objective methods and standards. Standards and criteria must be established and accepted, readily applied and observable in product or in process.

Evaluation can be conducted by the use of check lists, rating scales, questionnaires, inventories, tests, observation and work measurement on the job. Results can be measured by external criteria such as: absenteeism, break-in time for new hires, patient complaints, employee attitudes, grievances, work stoppages, sick-leave usage, turnover, pool of promotable men and budget fulfillment.

Certain other principles of evaluation have been suggested: [22]

1. Decisions about evaluation should be an integral part of the planning phase of the program design.

2. Evaluation should contain an element of measurement.

3. Evaluation should follow a systematic design.

The evaluation process is an integral part of the training and development responsibility. In identifying training needs and planning training programs, the personnel administrator must incorporate a method for evaluating results. This method cannot be a one-shot program but must be ongoing, moving into a systematic follow-up plan for the improvement and modification of the training program.

Notes

1. Bleick Von Bleicken, *Employee Training Handbook* (Philadelphia: Chilton Company, 1953), p. 13.

2. Addison C. Bennett, "Can Hospitals Afford Not to Have a Training Program?" *Hospitals* (December 16, 1967), p. 59.

3. *Idem.*

4. "American Hospital Association Statement on the Coordination of Education and Training Programs," *Hospitals* (January 16, 1968), pp. 121-2.

5. Paul M. Stokes, *Total Job Training* (New York: American Management Association, 1966), pp. 16-19.

6. George D. Halsey, *Training Employees* (New York: Harper and Bros., 1949), p. 2.

7. George S. Odiorne, *Personnel Policy: Issues and Practices* (Columbus, O.: Charles E. Merrill Books, Inc., 1963), p. 244.

8. James M. Black and Guy B. Ford, *Front-Line Management* (New York: McGraw-Hill Book Company, 1963), pp. 135-8.

9. Carl R. Rogers, "Centennial Conference on Communications: Northwestern University, 1951," *Harvard Business Review* (July-August, 1952).

10. The material in this section was developed with the assistance of Dr. Leslie Slote, Management Psychologist, Hartsdale, New York.

11. Chris Argyris, *Interpersonal Competence and Organizational Effectiveness* (Homewood, Ill.: Richard D. Irwin, Inc., The Dorsey Press, Inc., 1962); pp. 134-9.

12. Kurt W. Back, "Sensitivity Training: Questions and Quest," *Personnel Administration* (January-February, 1971), p. 22.

13. For a discussion of this subject, see *Harvard Business Review* (July-August, 1970), pp. 150-67.

14. Much of the material in this section was developed by Miller-Ginsburg Associates, 462 Germantown Pike, LaFayette Hill, Pennsylvania.

15. Robert L. Desatnick, *A Concise Guide to Management Development* (New York: American Management Association, 1970), p. 11.

16. Walter S. Wikstrom, *Supervisory Training* (New York: The Conference Board, Inc., 1943), pp. 1-16.

17. *Idem.*

18. *Idem.*

19. *Idem.*

20. *Training and Continuing Education: A Handbook for Health Care Institutions* (Chicago: Hospital Research & Education Trust, 1970).

21. William R. Travey, *Evaluating Training and Development Systems* (New York: American Management Association, 1968), pp. 14-15.

22. *Training and Continuing Education, op. cit.,* pp. 223-4.

VII. UNION ORGANIZATIONAL DRIVES: PREVENTIVE LABOR RELATIONS*

> To convince unorganized workers that they need unionism requires know-how, a thorough knowledge of the individual worker's job and his role in producing the company's product, and a certain interest in the worker's specific problems.
>
> The impersonal approach cannot get the organizer's message over to unorganized workers; it can never take the place of person-to-person contact, nor can it cope with the tactics developed by anti-union employers. Management as we know, has recognized the importance of building up individual relationships with its employees—through supervisors and foremen. Organizers cannot hope to be successful until their own relationship with the workforce is strong enough to overcome management's campaign to develop union hostility.[1]

The preceding quotation is the advice of a union official to a union organizer in an official guidebook published by the union. It would appear that the key to a successful organizing program, as the union views it, is a personalized campaign which relates to the individual employee's problems. Now what about the administration's "campaign"?

Angelo Patri, a well-known educator and renowned expert on child development, was reported to have answered a mother who asked him, "When should I begin teaching my six-month-old son the way to behave?," "Madam, you are already six months too late." When a health care facility administrator requests information on preventive labor relations after a union has petitioned for recognition, any expert in the field would state, "Sir, you are already six months too late." The time for preventive labor relations—that is, for implementing sound personnel policies—is before employees look to the *outside* for the answer to unsolved needs. Simply stated, preventive labor relations is the science of providing an atmosphere

---

*Reprinted, with permission, from Chapter II, "Preventive Labor Relations," *Labor Relations and Personnel Management in Long-Term Health Care Facilities* by Norman Metzger and Dennis D. Pointer, Ph.D. (Washington, D.C.: American Health Care Association, 1975), pp. 3-8.
Note: The phrase "nursing home" in the original text has been changed to "health care facility" or "institution."

in the health care facility which recognizes the dignity of the employee and rewards employees in relation to their efforts toward the final goal of the health care facility: providing sound care.

A health care facility which provides all the protections afforded employees in a unionized institution will rarely become organized. *Unions do not organize health care facility employees, but rather health care facility employees are driven into unions by poor administrative practices.* In the final analysis more employees vote for or against their immediate supervisors than vote for or against their institution. Therefore, preventive labor relations must focus on the first line of defense for the institution, supervisors and department heads.

Is Union Organization of Employees in Your Institution Inevitable?

Although it is a fact that in the health services industry unions win almost half the elections, the answer to the question—Is union organization of your employees inevitable?—depends on the organizational life-style that administration has built up over the years in the institution. The key to maintaining an institution's nonunion status and, indeed, the key to maintaining a highly efficient and productive institution, is the first-line supervisor. The supervisor as communicator (or noncommunicator) is the essential ingredient. Marrihue tells us of a culture existing in one of the small islands of the Samoan group.[2] Upon this island, which is a tiny protype of a highly complex industrial society, all men are chiefs. The women do all the work. But there are two types of chiefs: the regular chiefs who are powerless, but who are in the majority, and the *talking* chiefs who run the island!

We can spend time extensively outlining the supervisor's activities and earmarking special skills which they must bring to the work situation, but in the final analysis, the mark of the successful supervisor is the ability to communicate. What separates the supervisor from the worker is the fact that the person in a supervisory position must get work done through *other* people and, to accomplish this, must communicate effectively with them.

If a health care facility can build up a climate of trust and confidence, its side of the story will have enormous effect when and if the union enters the scene. In the long run employees are influenced not by what the administration of a facility says, but by what it does.

Unions in general often display superior communication skills compared with those of administration. They seem to have an uncanny ability to anticipate employees' moods, problems and priorities. The key to their overall strategy is to put the administration on the defensive in its (administration's) attempts to communicate with employees: so an institution may spend its idle hours responding to leaflets, answering charges and defending its past record.

The time to win employee loyalty and confidence is before the union starts its organization drive. Any actions that the administration of a health care facility may take during the organizational campaign are far less important when compared to the overall record of that administration during the preceding years. That is not to say that the administration's campaign is unimportant to the final outcome of a certification election, but rather that it is less important than the effect of poor personnel practices that may have been part of the record of employee-management relations over the years. Such practices as low wages, substandard fringe benefits, favoritism and poor supervision are more likely to override any positive effects of a management campaign when the union arrives on the scene.

Communications: The Key to Employee Loyalty

Although employees are more impressed by what the administration does than by what the administration says, it has been determined that communication is the key to winning employee loyalty. The real payoff in communication comes through the art of listening. In many cases where unions are successful in their attempts to organize homes, it has been found that the employees of those institutions felt that the health care facility was totally unconcerned with them as individuals. Employees turn to unionization when their needs are not fulfilled. Employee needs are not fulfilled when the administration does not listen carefully and sensitively to what the employees are saying.

The core of the problem of supervisory communication is the misconception about the art and basic components of good communications. Too many supervisors think that communication is a one-way street with such signs as "Tell," "Inform," and "Order." The absence of an appreciation of the other elements of communication such as "Listening," "Asking," and "Interpreting" is central to the failure in communication. Very often fear, suspicion or jealousy nullifies the sense of the words used by the supervisor. The supervisor should ask himself six questions before attempting to communicate with his employees:

1. Do I assume that if an idea is clear to me it will be clear to the receiver?

2. Do I make it comfortable for others to tell me what is really on their minds . . . or do I encourage them to tell me only what I like to hear?

3. Do I check my understanding of what another person has told me before I reply?

4. Am I tolerant of other people's feelings, realizing that their feelings, which may be different from mine, affect their communication?

5. Do I really try to listen from the sender's point of view before evaluating the message from my point of view?

6. Do I make a conscious effort to build feedback possibility in all communications, since even at its best, communication is an imperfect process?

How Effective Is Your Preventive Labor Relations Program?

There are several means of judging the effectiveness of your employee relations efforts. Blai suggests the following: comments of workers, actions of management and supervision, and records.[3] There are five specific records which may be used as points of comparison with comments of workers and actions of the administration:

1. *Quit rate.* The fact that many employees resign may have a significant relationship to the effectiveness of your personnel program and may indeed portend difficulty with the remaining employees.

2. *Grievances.* Of course, if there is no grievance mechanism or if the employee is apprehensive about the prospect of retaliatory reaction, such statistics alone are misleading, but they can indicate problem areas. It has been found that union organization usually starts in one department or on one shift. A careful analysis of where the problems (grievances) are centered will be very helpful in remedying such difficulties.

3. *Exit interviews.* Why do workers quit? An effective exit interview program with appropriate documentation can augment and cross-check turnover statistics and pinpoint deficiencies in personnel practices.

4. *Disciplinary actions.* One must be sensitive to the effectiveness of supervision before analyzing disciplinary action rates. Careful selection, training and motivation have an important influence on such statistics. It has been found that a concentration of disciplinary actions in one area or resulting from one type of offense can pinpoint potentially explosive situations which will lead to union organization.

5. *Sick leave utilization.* Taken along with other indicators, abuse of the sick leave benefit may reflect poor personnel policies or practices.

The best procedure is to establish a composite profile. The trend line should suggest whether your personnel efforts (preventive labor relations) have been successful or whether they need improvement.

Administrative Programs

There is no substitute for a well-trained, well-informed supervisor in the administration's effort to maintain a union-free institution. Selecting good supervisors and training those supervisors is not an easy job. In addition to training new supervisors, the administration must continuously retrain present supervisors and bring to them up-to-date methods in dealing with employee relations. Supervisors should be trained in the following elements:

1. How to discuss simple gripes and complaints.
2. How to deal with rumors.
3. How to explain rules and policies.
4. How to choose the means and manner of communication which best fit specific situations.
5. How to choose the means and manner of communication which best fit any situation.
6. How to communicate the administration's objectives to the workers; how to convince them of the importance of such objectives.

To an administrator of a health care facility, training and developing supervisors is inescapable . . . not just a "single" "short-term," "one-shot" or "booster" type program . . . but a continuing effort, a variety of programs and, most typical of the successful experiences in training, one with professional leadership and planning. It is well to note that most supervisors learn their style of management from their immediate boss. It is, therefore, essential to develop an organizational life-style which encourages supervisors toward good employee relations practices.

A Checklist: How Effective Is Your Program?

Too often administration gives little attention and little support to the establishment of a professional personnel department. The preoccupation of administrators and trustees in financial, construction and medical program matters leaves little or no time available to focus attention on an employee relations agenda. Too late the cry is heard, "why are our employees organizing?". It is not a fortuitous occurance, but one that is predictable: the box score of vulnerability is easily constructed. As the television commercial says: "See me now, or see me later". Either a committment is made in advance to build a strong personnel program, or one will-per-force be needed when the union is on the scene. The collective bargaining agreement is often a codification of many sound personnel matters; if such practices were in place before the union came around, the institution may well have remained non-union!

How do you measure the success of your personnel department? The keys to such an evaluation lie in a checklist to which every administrator of a health care facility should from time to time refer and rate for performance as against expectations:

1. Personnel Policy Manual:
    a. When was it written?
    b. When was it revised?
    c. Does it contain the entire statement of policy operative for all levels of personnel?

2. Job Evaluation Program:
    a. Are all jobs evaluated?
    b. Are all jobs described?
    c. Have you developed a wage and salary program?
    d. Is it competitive and up to date?
    e. Are increases based upon clearly understood criteria?

3. Orientation and Induction Program:
    a. Do you have one?
    b. Are all new employees included in it?
    c. Is there a follow-up after the probationary period?

4. Performance Evaluation Program:
    a. Are all employees evaluated at least once a year?
    b. Are the evaluations discussed with the individual employee?
    c. Do employees know what is expected of them?

5. Training Program:
    a. Is there an opportunity for present employees to improve their skills through training?
    b. Is training a continuing function or a one-shot operation?
    c. Do you have an ongoing supervisory development program?

6. Have you control over your Employee Benefits Program?
    a. Do you know the costs of your benefits?
    b. Do you have a broad package of benefits competitive with other health care facilities and industries in your area?
    c. Are your eligibility requirements clearly defined and in writing?
    d. Do you have a regular review of your benefits package?

7. Staffing Controls:
    a. Is the approval mechanism for positions clearly defined?
    b. Do you have carefully researched and evaluated recruitment sources?
    c. Do you hire on the basis of an application form; interview; test; reference check?
    d. Do you follow up placements after a probationary period?

e. Do you maintain turnover records?

f. Do you evaluate costs of recruitment?

g. Do you analyze vacancies to ascertain whether jobs should be filled after specific period of time of vacancy?

h. Do you have a monthly report on the Table of Organization containing authorized positions and filled positions in each department of the facility?

8. Do you have a formalized employee relations program?

a. Can employees bring their grievances to someone outside of their department?

b. Can grievances which are not settled inside the facility be arbitrated by an outside individual?

c. Do you have a counseling service for employees' nonjob-connected problems?

d. Do you have a tuition refund program to encourage employees to further their education?

e. Do you have an awards program to recognize long-term employees' service?

f. Do you have a house organ with human interest stories about employees and facility activities?

9. Is your personnel administrator doing ongoing research as to what other institutions and industrial firms are doing in the field of personnel and employee relations?

If you score high on this checklist, you will have no concern over unionization. Unions do not appear where an institution has a planned, positive and progressive personnel program.

A Nonunion-Oriented Grievance Procedure

The burden of a grievance procedure is to bring employee complaints to the surface and to settle peacefully any disputes.[4] The grievance procedure is an integral part of the complete management communication network. If the mechanism that you develop to handle grievances is so cumbersome and works to discourage submission rather than encourage it, many unidentified and, of course, unsettled complaints will fester in their unresolved state and probably will develop into a crisis far out of perspective—indeed, much greater than the original problem.

In order to develop an appropriate grievance procedure in a nonunion environment, the following definition of a grievance must be accepted and embodied in the entire mechanism: a grievance exists when there is any employee discontent or dissatisfaction, whether valid or not, which arises out of anything connected with the institution that such employee thinks, believes or even feels is unfair, unjust or inequitable. Too often health care facility administrators avoid the introduction of a formal grievance mechanism because of the unfounded belief that such machinery invites grievances when, indeed, none really exist. This is a completely false assumption. Employees have problems and it is best to establish proper channels for reviewing such problems and adjudicating them. The idea that the "open door policy" and/or informal grievance procedure can substitute for a formal one has been proved ineffective and counterproductive. Most administrators find such activity to be an imposition on their busy schedules. This "open door policy" means that an employee must make an appointment, face a busy receptionist, enter an office which may be intimidating, and finally, confront an administrator with whom he has probably had little previous contact.

Good grievance machinery is important. Such machinery alone will not ensure success. The attitude, judgment, experience and training of the individual involved are of prime importance. Moreover, a desire to settle grievances rather than to win them is essential.[5]

A three-step grievance procedure would be most appropriate for the average health care facility. At the first step, the employee would present the grievance to the immediate supervisor. Such grievance meetings should be permitted during working hours, but the final decision as to the specific time for presentation of the grievance should be at the sole discretion of the supervisor based upon patient needs or work schedules. Caveat: if an employee believes that the presentation of the grievance is an urgent matter, be sensitive to such feelings. It is not necessary for the employee to formalize the grievance in writing at this initial stage.

Although time is of the essence, haste is counterproductive to the adjudication of employee grievances. The supervisor should be sensitive to the need for taking as much time as necessary to determine, *through investigations,* the material facts of the grievance. The first-line supervisor's response to the first-step grievance presentation should be made within three to five working days. If extra time is necessary, the supervisor should inform the aggrieved employee of the need and the reason for the extension of time in answering the grievance.

When the supervisor is prepared to respond to the grievance, the employee should be given a complete and clear answer. If the employee accepts the answer and does not intend to appeal to the next step, the supervisor should make anecdotal notes of the settlement of the grievance and keep such notes in departmental files. If the employee is dissatisfied with the response and intends to appeal, the supervisor should present the details of the grievance and the response in writing and forward the written reports to the next step.

The second step of the grievance procedure would have the aggrieved employee appealing the decision of his first-line supervisor to either a department head or a personnel director. Again, time should be arranged during working hours for the employee to present his grievance at this step. Once again, a reply should be presented to the employee within three to five working days from the time of the hearing. Records of the response should be kept in writing. The employee should have the option to accept the decision at the second step or appeal to the third and final step.

A third-step appeal could be made to an associate administrator or a personnel director if the latter individual was not part of the second step. A similar procedure to the first and second steps would be followed. Two controversial elements must be discussed at this point if proper consideration is to be given to the establishment of a nonunion grievance procedure.

First, the possibility of representation for the employee at each of the steps of the grievance procedure should be considered. Employees can be given the opportunity to select another employee as their spokesman in the presentation of grievances. Some employees may not be comfortable in presenting grievances and will find it more acceptable to have other employees speak for them. The opportunity to select a fellow employee to present the grievance presents a further image of fairness on the part of the institution.

Second, the availability of arbitration of unsettled grievances outside the institution should be considered. It has been said that effective grievance adjustment requires establishment of voluntary arbitration by a disinterested party as a terminal step in the grievance machinery. Most institutions prefer to guard their management prerogatives and do not look kindly on the imposition of "second guessing" by parties outside their institution. Notwithstanding the inherent negatives, serious thought should be given to the possibility of establishing an avenue of recourse outside the institution as the final step in the grievance procedure. This could very well be the selection of a respected member of the community, a respected member of the clergy in the community, or a professor in one of the local colleges. If the administration of the home dislikes such a mechanism, an alternative would be the presentation of the employee's grievance to a member or a committee of the board of directors.

Two variations on the suggestions above are indeed worth serious consideration. Some nonunion grievance procedures include the provision of assistance by a member of the personnel department in submitting an employee's grievance. This assistance replaces a fellow employee representative and casts the personnel department representative in the role of ombudsman. This procedure would preclude the personnel department from being a part of the management structure in the grievance procedure. A second variation for consideration is the availability of the director or administrator of the health care facility as the final step in the grievance procedure. In many instances this opportunity to present the grievance to the director at the final step will substitute for the need for outside arbitration.[6]

Why Employees of Health Care Facilities Join Unions and What to Do About It

Many attempts at organizing employees of health care facilities center on wages. Yet more often than not, employee dissatisfaction centers on nonfinancial elements. Employees look to unions because:

1. They are not receiving appropriate recognition.
2. There are only limited avenues for promotion.
3. They feel a lack of respect for their dignity in the institution.
4. There is no avenue for *participation;* they are not consulted regarding changes which affect them.
5. There is no mechanism for bringing grievances to satisfactory adjudication.
6. There is a lack of communication between employees and the employer.
7. There are unfavorable working conditions.
8. Supervisors are unsympathetic, arrogant and disinterested.

To permit these conditions to fester and remain unsolved is a direct invitation to unionization. The administration of health care facilities must listen to their employees and pinpoint areas of concern—real concern. Simply listening to the problems of employees through formal and informal mechanisms is often half the solution to the problem. A complete two-way communications program must be instituted. Such programs which are successful incorporate the use of house organs, employee policy handbooks, bulletin board notices, letters to the home and scheduled meetings between administration and rank-and-file employees.

Once the union does appear on the scene, much thought must be given to the area of communication within the context of a campaign. Although the legal distinction between permissible campaigning and unfair labor practices is at times difficult to make, the following checklist of actions an administrator can take and cannot take in this period is offered:[7]

The health care facility can:

1. Explain the meaning of union recognition and the procedure to be followed.

2. Encourage each member of the bargaining unit to vote in the election.

3. Communicate to employees that they are free to vote for or against the union notwithstanding the fact that they signed a union authorization card.

4. Communicate to all employees the reasons why the administration is against recognizing a union.

5. Review the compensation and benefits program, pointing out the record of the administration in the past.

6. Point out to employees statements which the union has made which the administration believes to be untrue; communicate its own position on each of these statements.

7. If there is a general "no solicitation" rule which has been scrupulously adhered to, prevent solicitation of membership by the union during working hours.

8. Enforce all rules and regulations in effect prior to the union's request for recognition, if they have been enforced in the past.

9. Carefully prepare and distribute letters to employees' homes stating the administration's position and record and the administration's knowledge of the union's position in other hospitals.

10. Point out the possibility of strikes when unions enter health care facilities and their ramifications.

11. Discuss the impact of union dues and all costs surrounding membership in a union.

12. Highlight to employees the fact that a union can promise employees anything, but it can only deliver on promises with the agreement of administration.

13. Hold individual discussions with employees at their work area to communicate the position of the institution.

14. As union promises are communicated to employees during the preelection period, point out to the employees that if the health care facility is to meet such demands, it might be forced to lay off workers.

The health care facility cannot and should not:

1. Make promises of benefits and threats of reprisals if the employees vote against the union or for the union; have supervisors attend union meetings; spy on the activities of the employees to determine whether they are participating in union activities.

2. Grant wage increases or special concessions during the preelection period unless the timing coincides with well-established prior practices.

3. Prevent employees from wearing union buttons, except in cases where the buttons are provocative or extremely large.

4. Bar employee-union representatives from soliciting employee membership during nonworking hours when the solicitation does not interfere with the work of others.

5. Summon an employee into an office to privately discuss the union and the upcoming election.

6. Question employees about union matters and meetings.

7. Attempt to ascertain from an employee how he intends to vote.

8. Threaten employees with layoffs due to unionization or state that the institution will never deal with the union even if it is certified.

To do nothing or to remain neutral when the union appears is the surest way to become organized. To overreact or to change your policies, procedures and general employee relations programs may be both misinterpreted by your employees and be deemed unfair labor practices by the National Labor Relations Board. The soundest approach is a carefully planned, sensitive and believable program which has as its cornerstone, *your supervisors.*

Notes

1. Nicholas Zonarich, *Introduction to A Guidebook for Union Organizers*, Industrial Union Department, AFL-CIO.
2. Willard V. Merrihue, *Managing by Communication* (New York: McGraw-Hill Book Company, 1960), p. 4.
3. Boris Blai, Jr., "How Effective Is Your Personnel Program?," *Personnel Journal*, Vol. 30, No. 3 (July-August, 1951), pp. 21-2.
4. C. W. Randle and M. F. Wortman, Jr., *Collective Bargaining Principles and Practices* (New York: Houghton-Mifflin Co., 1966), p. 227.
5. Frank Elkouri and Edna Asper Elkouri, *How Arbitration Works*, 3rd edition (Washington, D.C.: Bureau of National Affairs, Inc., 1973), p. 110.
6. See Chapter VIII, for further discussions of grievance procedures.
7. A committee of the American Bar Association and a committee of publishers and associates included in a declaration of principles that writers who deal with any subject that has or may have legal overtones shall declare that they are not engaged in rendering legal services. *If legal service or other expert assistance is required, the services of a competent professional should be sought.*

VIII. CONTRACT ADMINISTRATION: THE GRIEVANCE AND ARBITRATION PROCEDURES*

The Negotiated Grievance Procedure

> ". . . the collective bargaining agreement states the rights and duties of the parties; it is a generalized code to govern a myriad of cases which the draftsmen cannot wholly anticipate. It calls into being a new common law . . ."[1]

This common law, referred to by Mr. Justice Douglas, includes a grievance procedure. It has been said that no other phase of the labor-management relationship provides the management with greater opportunity to win employee respect and confidence than the grievance procedure.[2] Conversely, an expert observer of unionism in our country states flatly that the handling of workers' grievances on the job is perhaps the single most important function of modern unionism.[3]

A very parochial view of collective bargaining sees that process terminating at the signing of a contract. This is an invalid construction of the process. The cold, hard language of this contract must be transfused into a living, breathing mechanism. The procedure designed to do just that is the grievance procedure.

To begin with, just what is a *grievance?* A grievance exists when there is any employee "discontent or dissatisfaction, whether valid or not," which arises out of "anything connected with the" hospital that such employee "thinks, believes, or even feels is unfair, unjust or inequitable."

The burden of a *grievance procedure,* then, "is to bring employee complaints to the surface and to settle peacefully any disputes."[4]

It is an integral part of a management communication network. If the mechanism that you develop to handle grievances is so cumbersome, and works to discourage submission rather than encourage it, then many unidentified and, of course, unsettled complaints will fester in their unresolved

*Reprinted, with permission, from *Hospitals, Journal of the American Hospital Association,* Vol. 48 (April 16, 1974), pp. 47-9; and (May 1, 1974), pp. 45-7.

state, and most probably develop into a crisis far out of perspective, and indeed much greater than the original problem.

Yet too often, administrators avoid the establishment of formal grievance procedures because of a misguided belief that such machinery invites grievances where none existed. Grievance machinery or not, your employees have problems. Still another fallacy, indeed a rationalization, is the substitution of an informal grievance procedure for a formal one. Can an employee at a lower level truly express his frustrations, his fears, his needs to a person in a much higher position who appears to him to be isolated from the everyday problems of the working man? Is it not true that many executives find such activity to be an imposition on their busy schedules? The employee must make an appointment; he must pass through a receptionist who often is protective as to her boss' time; he must enter into an office which at times is large, formal and foreboding. Then he must face a man who he might never have talked to in the year before and probably will never talk to in the year ahead; and at this point one expects him to talk and argue freely. This is why the structure of the grievance procedure is so vital to its success.

The structure of the negotiated grievance procedure varies greatly as to the degree of complexity and formality. In formalizing the grievance procedure when a union enters the hospital, the following basic points must be considered and appropriate decisions made which will produce a facile and productive mechanism:

1. What constitutes a grievance?
2. What is the procedure for submitting a grievance?
3. How many steps will constitute the procedure?
4. Who will be present at each step for both sides?
5. What time limits will be invoked in presenting and answering the grievance?
6. Will employees and steward be paid for time spent in making use of the grievance procedure?

A far more limited and prevalent scope of the grievance procedure refers to a grievance as a difference of opinion between management and an employee or the union specifically relating to the *meaning and application* of the terms of the collective bargaining agreement. This would reduce and limit the arbitrator's role to one of a judicial rather than legislative nature; his objective would be to interpret the already bargained positions of the parties.

One might look at grievance-handling from two different vantage points; the clinical and the legalistic. The legalistic approach emphasizes form and mechanics. It directs its attention to accepting or dismissing grievances on the basis of whether or not they are within the contract. The clinical approach attempts to get to the heart of the problem. This approach is advocated by Benjamin M. Selikman.[5] He recommends the intensive search for the fundamental determinants of a grievance rather than accepting at face value its surface rationale. This method bespeaks of an empathetic probe into the actual circumstances and causes of the grievance. Actually the latter approach can augment the former, and indeed the two approaches are not mutually exclusive.

There are four basic principles of grievance adjustment. These principles were outlined by Van D. Kennedy as follows:[6]

1. Grievances should be adjusted promptly, preferably at the first step in the grievance procedure, and the adjustment of grievances should be on their merits. The overwhelming majority of grievances can and should be informally adjusted and disposed of at the *foreman-steward* level.

2. The machinery for submission of a grievance must be easy to utilize and well-understood both by the worker and his supervisor.

3. Regardless of the particular mechanical details or number of steps in the procedure, it is essential that the need for a direct avenue of appeal from the rulings of line supervision be recognized.

4. Effective grievance adjustment requires establishment of voluntary arbitration by a disinterested party as the terminal step in the contract's grievance machinery.

Broadly speaking, management's responsibility for grievance procedure administration embraces three primary functions:

1. Investigating the material facts of grievances.

2. Discussing and answering grievances.

3. Analyzing grievances to determine the basic causes.

The union's responsibility for grievance procedure participation embraces:

1. Discussing and investigating grievance facts with employee.

2. Presenting grievance to management.

3. Appeal of grievance through various steps of grievance procedure.

If grievance administrators are to discharge their grievance handling responsibilities properly, their first task upon receiving a grievance is to *investigate—not evaluate.*[7]

In the adjustment of grievances, as in so many other aspects of labor relations, time is of the essence. That's why it is customary for each step in the procedure to carry with it a time limit, at the expiration of which the dispute goes to the next stage. Management usually wants to be protected from grievances arising out of events long past. For this reason, the right to initiate grievances under many contracts is conditioned upon the presentation being made within a specified number of days following the event or incident precipitating the grievance.

Not only management, however, is concerned with the prompt handling of grievances. The union and its members, too, justifiably want and deserve safeguards against possible oversight or neglect of grievances by management. To prevent this, many grievance procedures expressly specify time limits within which management representatives, at each step of the procedure, must answer grievances. Where such provisions exist and the management representative fails to answer the grievance within the prescribed time limits, some contracts further provide that the grievance shall be settled on the basis of the relief sought in the grievance. In other contracts, the union simply is free to advance the grievance to the next higher step. Adequate opportunity for proper investigation and review of grievances should not be sacrificed simply to permit the speedy processing of grievances.

Unlike the matter of time limits, the extent to which the employer should bear the cost of time spent by employees on grievance activity can become a controversial bargaining issue. Management quite naturally views this question from the cost impact due to lost time and the loss in direct operating costs. Unions maintain that pay for such activity should be absorbed by the employer as he would any other item of normal overhead expense. Under most contracts today, the aggieved employee himself is paid for time lost from work in the processing of his own grievance. Similarly, it is fairly common practice to pay shop stewards and a specified number of grievance committeemen.

In determining what grievance activity is to be paid for, contracts sometimes distinguish between time spent *investigating* grievances and that spent actually *adjusting* them. Where such distinctions are made, some companies pay only for time spent adjusting grievances, but allow time without pay for the investigation of grievances or do not permit the investigation during working hours.

Limitations on the amount of grievance time to be paid for by the employer vary widely. Some contracts specify a flat number of company-paid hours per contract year for grievance activity. Others provide similar limits, but on a daily, weekly or monthly basis. Still others provide control by limiting the number of persons to be paid at any step of the procedure.

With the advent of a formal, negotiated grievance procedure, there is introduced into the hospital a new level of employee, the shop steward. The shop steward often is aggressive, obdurate and militant, and will, in the case of prerogatives abdicated by the foreman, fill the vacuum left between supervisor and the employees. The supervisor is hard-pressed to consider the shop steward as a legitimate extension of the employee's voice; at times he (the steward) appears stentorian in his presentation.

The supervisor has the following six responsibilities in handling grievances:

1. Hearing the complaint.
2. Getting the facts.
3. Making the decision.
4. Communicating the decision.
5. Preparing a written record.
6. Minimizing grievances.

The possibility of having his decision reversed at a later step in the grievance procedure is one that must be dealt with realistically. It behooves the first-line supervisor to consult with higher administrative levels and the labor relations staff to not only assure consistency in contract administration, but to hedge against the possibility of a reversal. In the face of such possibility, the supervisor must be prepared to follow the rules of the game to ensure a firm and correct decision. What follows is a checklist of actions to take when handling a grievance:

1. Listen—permit the presentation of the full story by the employee and/or the steward.

2. Try to understand—keep prodding with how, who, what, when, where and why.

3. Separate fact from emotion—take the time to *investigate.*

4. Refer to policy and contract provisions—never forget that a supervisor cannot offer a solution or make an agreement which is contrary to the provisions of the collective bargaining agreement.

5. Remember that your decision may set a precedent—if you decide to interpret a clause of the contract loosely, it may set a precedent for all other similar cases.

6. Consult with others—check with other supervisors who may have had a similar grievance; check with the personnel department.

7. Explain your decision fully—avoid curt remarks, but be explicit and honest in communicating your decision.

All grievances should be heard whether they are covered by the definition in the contract or not. To protect the contractual relationship, a compromise between the clinical and the legalistic interpretation of the procedure may easily be drawn by limiting the types of grievances which may be referred to arbitration. This could be simply stated by defining as arbitrable issues those which involve a question of contract interpretation or application.

It would seem abundantly clear that the formalizing of the grievance procedure as a result of a collective bargaining agreement would put the added burden of documentation onto the shoulders of supervision. Whether or not the union appeared on the scene, the need for a grievance procedure has been clearly established. All that is added into the bag of administrative tools is a clear and orderly system of remitting of the facts regarding grievances to writing.

The Arbitration Procedure

Provisions for the use of arbitration to resolve disputes during the life of a contract appear in well over 90 percent of all collective bargaining agreements. In a study made of major collective bargaining agreements by the U.S. Department of Labor, it was found that 1,609 of the 1,717 agreements studied had provisions for arbitration.[8]

Further, the proportion of agreements providing for grievance arbitration has increased steadily.

The arbitration of disputes between management and labor has been hailed as a means of ensuring uninterrupted operations. It is intended as a substitute for work stoppages and strikes. Practitioners in the field believe that, in terms of any particular clause of the contract, the arbitration provision is sometimes the only positive advantage that management is able to obtain in its negotiations with a union.

Slichter stated over 30 years ago that industrial relations had developed into industrial jurisprudence, which follows a system of law and legal procedure that clearly labels the practice of labor relations as judicial.[9] Arbitration is a lawful technique for resolving disputes between management and a union that evolve during the life of the contract. Kagel hoists several red flags that should be acknowledged at the outset of any protracted discussion of the arbitration technique:

1. The best way to settle a dispute—any dispute—is by negotiation. Most disputes are in fact settled in this way.

2. Arbitration should be the last resort of the parties in the same way that courts should be used as a last resort in a legal controversy.

3. Arbitration should never be used as a substitute for negotiations, nor should it be used, except in rare instances, as a device to "save face."[10]

The Legal Framework

Voluntary arbitration as a terminal step in the grievance procedure has a long history. It was put on firm footing by several decisions of the U.S. Supreme Court starting in 1957. In the *Lincoln Mills* case in 1957 the Court held that Section 301(a) of the Labor Management Relations Act empowers the federal courts to compel specific performance of arbitration clauses in collective bargaining agreements and that the federal courts should direct arbitration where, generally speaking, they found both a nonstrike clause and an arbitration clause in an agreement.[11] Three decisions handed down in 1960, commonly called the "trilogy," furthered the cause of arbitration in labor disputes. In the first case, *Warrior and Gulf Navigation,* the Court ruled that a specific dispute could be arbitrated unless the parties specifically excluded the subject of the dispute from the arbitration process.[12] In the second case, *American Manufacturing Company,* the Court held that federal courts are limited in determining whether a dispute is covered by a labor agreement and are not authorized to evaluate the merits of the dispute—the courts could not consider the merits of a grievance, only whether it is covered by the contract.[13] In the third case, *Enterprise Wheel and Car Corporation,* the Court ruled that the interpretation of a collective bargaining agreement is a question for arbitration, not for the court.[14] That is, an arbitrator's award that is within the scope of the contract must be enforced whether or not the courts agree with his interpretation.

Differences between Judicial and Legislative Arbitration
Voluntary arbitration as the terminal step of a grievance procedure in contract administration disputes is judicial in nature. Judicial arbitration is the prevalent form of labor arbitration in the United States. When a union and a hospital or nursing home are unable to resolve a dispute by mutual agreement, by provision by the contract the parties can submit the particular issue to an impartial third party for solution. Such an arbitrator may not amend, modify, add to or delete any term of the agreement. The arbitrator's authority is limited to interpreting and applying some term of the collective bargaining agreement. His decision is final and binding on both parties. His authority is clearly outlined in the contract; he is much like a judge who is called upon to interpret a breach of contract lawsuit. This form of arbitration is the terminal point of the grievance procedure in most collective bargaining agreements.

Legislative arbitration, on the other hand, authorizes the arbitrator to write or rewrite contract langue that is in dispute. An arbitrator in this instance usually receives his authority from a law, and he is called upon to be a policymaking individual. This form of arbitration is rarely found in labor relations in the United States. It is used at the time of an impasse in reaching the terms of an agreement, while judicial arbitration is usually limited to disputes evolving from contract interpretation during the life of the contract.

The negotiation of a contract provision for the process of arbitration must address itself to three major questions:

1. Shall the arbitrator be selected on an ad hoc basis or a permanent basis?

2. Shall there be a single arbitrator or an arbitration panel?

3. Which issues shall be permitted to go to arbitration?

Type of Arbitrator

Most contract provisions for arbitration defer the selection of the arbitrators to the time of the dispute. When an issue is in dispute, the parties jointly select an arbitrator. This ad hoc selection of a separate arbitrator for each issue (although the parties may select the same man more than one time for other issues) has the marked advantage of securing a qualified individual to rule on a particular type of dispute. The parties will look for a qualified arbitrator who has had experience ruling on the particular type of issue in dispute. The permanent arbitrator provision is less widely used in the United States. Under this method, both parties mutually select an impartial arbitrator to handle all arbitrations during the life of the specific agreement. This has the advantage of providing the parties with a carefully selected individual who has earned the respect of both labor and management and who, because of repeated experience with the parties, can develop a thorough understanding of the problems and unique difficulties of a particular institution.

Single Arbitrator vs. Panel

Provision for the use of a single arbitrator appointed for each case was found in 42 percent of contracts studied by the U.S Department of Labor, while provision for an ad hoc arbitration panel was specified in 39 percent of the contracts. The most common type of panel is one composed of an equal number of management and union representatives who together choose an impartial member who acts as chairman. It has been stated that a decision rendered by a tripartite board—composed of one member elected by the union, one selected by management, and one impartial individual—ultimately reduces decision-making to the choice of the impartial member. Using a single arbitrator or an arbitration panel composed entirely of impartial individuals to resolve disputes arising from the contract appears to be the most effective approach to arbitration.

What Shall Be Arbitrated?

Under voluntary arbitration provisions in a labor contract, the arbitrator's authority stems from the mutually agreed upon definition incorporated in the contract. The parties must have agreed to make arbitration the final step in the solution of any dispute in order for the arbitrator to assume authority. The contract may indeed make certain disputes non-arbitrable. It is important to recognize that the arbitrator's authority stems only from the contract language. He cannot extend his authority beyond that prescribed by contract language. It is not unusual for the parties to proscribe certain disputes from the arbitration procedure. In the case of hospitals and nursing homes, contracts may limit the arbitration procedure to matters not involving patient care.

In negotiating a clause providing for arbitration, the parties must be fully cognizant of the fact that an arbitrator exercises his authority through their agreement. It is well to note that if, in exercising his jurisdiction in an arbitration case, the arbitrator goes beyond the authority stated in the contract or submission agreement, his award can be voided. The hospital may want to exclude certain subjects, such as merit increases, promotions, introduction of new methods, and professional practices, from arbitration. It may do so by negotiating appropriate language in the contract.

Recent Developments

Davey pointed out that experience with the use of the arbitration procedure has produced several positive trends and developments.[15]

1. Marked improvement in understanding of proper uses of arbitration.

2. An increasing professionalization of the arbitration function.

3. A perceptible increase in the number of "permanent" arbitration relationships.

4. Definite improvement in contract clauses defining the grievance and arbitration procedures and the limits of arbitrable discretion.

5. Increased research interest in arbitration.

6. Development of new uses for arbitration as a method of determining interunion jurisdictional disputes and pension rights and also as an appellate procedure in union discipline cases.

7. Decline of the tripartite board in grievance disputes.

Davey also indicated certain questionable trends.

1. An observable tendency to exaggerate the precedential value of awards and to overlegalize the arbitration process.

2. Continued excessive use of arbitration in some relationships as a substitute for mature collective bargaining.

3. Inadequate use of arbitration decisions as instruments for training foremen and stewards in better contract administration.

4. Continued cynicism in some quarters, as shown by use of black-listing.

5. Continued deficiencies in the preparation and presentation of cases.

6. Inadequate screening procedures prior to arbitration.

The American Arbitration Association lists some common errors in arbitration.[16]

1. Using arbitration and arbitration costs as a harassing technique.

2. Overemphasis of the grievance by the union or exaggeration of an employee's fault by management.

3. Reliance on a minimum of facts and a maximum of arguments.

4. Concealing essential facts; distorting the truth.

5. Holding back books, records and other supporting documents.

6. Tying up proceedings with legal technicalities.

7. Introducing witnesses who have not been properly instructed on demeanor and on the place of their testimony in the entire case.

8. Withholding full cooperation from the arbitrator.

9. Disregarding the ordinary rules of courtesy and decorum.

10. Becoming involved in arguments with the other side. The time to try to convince the other party is before arbitration, during grievance processing. At the arbitration hearing, all efforts should be concentrated on convincing the arbitrator of the rightness of the hospital's position.

Unions and management have come to appreciate the value of arbitration and, concomitantly, its limitations. As a result of some hard experience, the contract clauses that specially provide for arbitration have been refined to indicate a clear mandate for the arbitrator. Research in arbitration has been aided by several services now available not only to the labor lawyers occupied in handling arbitration cases, but also to management. These include the Bureau of National Affairs, Commerce Clearing House, and the American Arbitration Association.

The American Arbitration Association

The American Arbitration Association (AAA) is probably most often used to provide arbitrators for disputes arising during the life of a collective bargaining agreement. It should be clear that no law or government agency mandates that the parties to a collective bargaining agreement use the AAA facilities. The parties, through negotiations, incorporate an arbitration clause and, in most cases, define the agency that shall provide the impartial arbitrators. Because most parties to collective bargaining agreements use ad hoc arbitration, it becomes necessary to select a mutually agreeable arbitrator for each case that is submitted to arbitration. In other words, the parties select an arbitrator for a specific case, without any commitment to use that arbitrator for any other dispute that might arise.

How Is the Arbitrator Selected?

Although legal training is obviously an advantage to an arbitrator, it does not follow that it is required that the arbitrator be a lawyer. Joseph Murphy, vice president of the AAA, points out that some of the best known arbitrators in the country are not lawyers and that the legal background necessary to adjudicate arbitration cases can be acquired without a law degree.

Louis Yagoda, a prominent arbitrator in the hospital field, states that many practitioners in the field have a prejudice against lawyers. Although he is not himself a lawyer, Mr. Yagoda would want the arbitrator to be a lawyer. He believes the arbitrator must have a legal background either by training or by exposure to the essentials of contract law.

Justice William O. Douglas, in writing the majority opinion in *Steelworkers v. Warrior and Gulf Navigation Company,* stated: "The labor arbitrator is usually chosen because of the parties' confidence in his knowledge of the common law of the shop and their trust in his personal judgment to bring to bear considerations which are not expressed in the contract as criteria for judgment. The parties expect that his judgment of a particular grievance will reflect not only what the contract says but, insofar as the collective bargaining agreement permits, such factors as the effect upon productivity of a certain result, its consequences to the morale of the shop; his judgment whether tensions will be heightened or diminished."

This seems to indicate the need for a professionally trained, legally equipped arbitrator who can interpret the contract and ascertain its intent. The American Arbitration Association has a simple and effective system for the selection of arbitrators. Upon receipt of the demand for arbitration, a copy of a list of proposed arbitrators is submitted to both parties. A short biographical sketch of each arbitrator on the list is attached. The tribunal administrator of the American Arbitration Association draws up this panel by considering the statement of the nature of the dispute submitted by the initiating party. The parties are then asked to indicate their preference by number, crossing out any names to which they object. This process of selection is done individually by the parties, and their lists are returned to the tribunal administrator, who attempts to match the union's preference with the employer's preference. If it is unable to establish a mutual choice on the list, the AAA submits additional lists. If the parties still cannot arrive at a mutual choice, the AAA makes an administrative appointment, but it never appoints a person whose name has been crossed off a list submitted to the parties.

Along with the biographical sketch of each arbitrator is an indication of his per diem fee. A little less than 17 percent of the arbitrators on the AAA panel charge less than $150. Approximately 40 percent charge $151-$200 per day, and approximately 3 percent charge more than $200 per day. These charges have recently gone up, obviously on the basis of inflation. In addition to the hearing day, arbitrators charge for study days, that is, time needed to review the case and arrive at a decision. The ratio of study days to hearing days is about 1.5 to 1, so that, on the average, the cost of arbitrating a case that can be heard in one day will be approximately $500. These costs are, in the main, shared equally by the parties. Such a provision to share costs is made part of the collective bargaining agreement.

How the Arbitration Case is Presented

The arbitration hearing is usually conducted in an informal atmosphere. Opening statements are made by each party. Usually, these statements are brief and are intended to identify the issue at dispute and suggest the relief that is sought. Many attorneys who represent employers will insist that the burden of proof is on the union because they have initiated the procedure and that, therefore, the union should be made to proceed first with its evidence. In itself, this is not a disadvantage. The right to present one's evidence first is generally considered an advantage and is given to the party that carries the burden of proof, partly to offset the disadvantages inherent in that burden but also partly because the logical method of proceeding is for the one who has advanced a grievance to state and to prove it.

The American Arbitration Association recommends that the opening statement be made orally, although some parties prefer to make it in writing. This statement often includes a stipulation of facts about the contract and of the circumstances surrounding the grievance. The presentation of evidence is an important part of the arbitration hearing.

While a certain degree of informality in the examination of witnesses is desirable, it must not interfere with the orderly presentation of the evidence. Witnesses are often the key to the presentation of facts. Every witness is subject to cross-examination, but the normal rules present in a court of law are not always obvious during the arbitration procedure. Arbitrators are not bound, as judges are, to apply the generally accepted rules of evidence. They may, and often do, receive any evidence, regardless of the rules, that seems important to an understanding of a case.

The introduction of documents as evidence is a most important part of the procedure. Although union attorneys often object to the introduction of employer documents (warning notices, written notes of events, performance evaluation forms, and the like), arbitrators normally will accept every piece of written documentation that seems to bear on the case. Each piece of documentary evidence is identified and numbered. Although arbitrators tend to accept documentary evidence, even though it is employer-initiated, the union lawyer has every right to object to the evidence if he considers it to be irrelevant. In most cases, the arbitrator will receive the evidence, or even testimony, that is objected to as irrelevant "for what it is worth."

Both parties are entitled to make closing statements. These statements include a summary of the factual situation and reiteration of the relief sought. The parties have the option to file written posthearing briefs. Posthearing briefs are usually discouraged, but should not be overlooked as a necessary element in presenting a highly technical case. The arbitrator will usually set a time limit on such submission.

Although erroneous rulings on evidence will not be grounds for attacking the validity of the award, unless they are so flagrant as clearly to indicate bias and unfairness, it would be highly improper and grounds for impeachment of the award if, after the hearing, the arbitrator should receive evidence from one side, *ex parte*.

Under AAA rules, the arbitrator has 30 days from the time that the hearing is closed to render his award, unless the collective bargaining agreement requires some other time limit. The award is made in writing and may be accompanied by an opinion discussing the evidence and setting forth the reasoning of the arbitrator. Some arbitrators maintain that the process could be speeded up if there was no need to support the award with an opinion. Still most parties prefer the clear delineation of the award by an opinion, which may well be educational in value.

Conclusion

The presentation of an arbitration case should not be left to amateurs. Although the atmosphere appears to be informal, the need for clear and professional presentation of the employer's case becomes obvious as the hearing moves on.

The Wisconsin Education Association has prepared guidelines on presenting arbitration cases.

1. Distinguish between what you know and what you can prove. Get proof. Interview all witnesses.

2. Hold a preparation conference in advance of the arbitration hearing. Plan how to offset the adversary's presentation.

3. Indicate to the witness how his story will help you. This will help the witness in cross-examination.

4. Stay away from uncertain witnesses.

5. Inspect all documentary evidence presented by the other side and also your own documentary evidence very carefully before allowing it to be entered as evidence to make sure it doesn't expand beyond your case.

6. In cross-examination, only ask those questions to which you know the answers.

7. Always try to convince the arbitrator, not the opposition.

Notes

1. Mr. Justice Douglas, *United Steelworkers of America v. Warrior and Gulf Navigation Company,* June 20, 1960.

2. Herron, Jr., *Negotiating and Administering the Grievance Procedure in Understanding Collective Bargaining,* American Management Association (New York, 1958).

3. Barbash, J., *The Practice of Unionism* (New York: Harper and Bros., 1956).

4. Randle, C. W. and Wortman, M. F., Jr., *Collective Bargaining Principles and Practice* (New York: Hougton-Mifflin Co., 1966).

5. Selikman, B. M., *Labor Relations and Human Relations* (New York: McGraw-Hill, 1947).

6. Kennedy, V. D., *Principles of Grievance Adjustment.*

7. Davey, H. W., *Contemporary Collective Bargaining,* 2nd edition (Englewood Cliffs, N.J.: Prentice-Hall, 1959).

8. U.S. Department of Labor, *Major Collective Bargaining Agreements: Grievance Procedures,* Bulletin 1425-6 (Washington, D.C.: U.S. Government Printing Office, June, 1966).

9. Slichter, S., *Union Policies and Industrial Management* (Washington, D.C.: Brookings Institution, 1941).

10. Kagel, S., *Anatomy of a Labor Arbitration* (Washington, D.C.: Bureau of National Affairs, 1961), p. ix.

11. *Textile Workers v. Lincoln Mills,* 353 US 448, 1957.

12. *United Steel Workers v. Warrior and Gulf Navigation Company,* U.S. Supreme Court, June 20, 1970.

13. *United Steel Workers v. American Manufacturing Company,* U.S. Supreme Court, June 20, 1970.

14. *United Steel Workers v. Enterprise Wheel and Car Corporation,* U.S. Supreme Court, June 20, 1970.

15. Davey, *op. cit.,* pp. 137-8.

16. *Labor Arbitration—Procedures and Techniques* (New York: American Arbitration Association, October, 1971).

ADDENDA

ADDENDUM A

The Mount Sinai Hospital Grievance Procedure
Part of the Collective Bargaining Agreement Between The Hospital
and District 1199, Drug and Hospital Employees Union, AFL-CIO

ARTICLE XXII—*Grievance Procedure*

Section A. A grievance is defined for purposes of this provision as a difference between the Hospital, and the Union, and/or an employee, concerning the interpretation and application of, or compliance with, any provision of this Agreement. When any such grievance arises, the following procedures shall be observed:

Step 1. An employee having a grievance may take it up directly with his supervisor or with his Department Steward, who shall take it up with the employee's supervisor.

A grievance of an employee may be presented either orally or in writing at this step of the grievance procedure. If the grievance is presented orally to the supervisor and is not satisfactorily settled, it must be promptly reduced to writing on the form provided.

When the grievance is reduced to writing, there shall be set forth in the spaces provided on the Grievance Form, the form of which is attached hereto in Appendix "D" all of the following:

a. Complete details of the grievance and the facts upon which it is based;

b. The remedy or correction which the grievant wishes the Hospital to make;

c. The grievance form shall be signed by the employee.

When the grievance is presented in writing, the answer of the supervisor shall be given in writing, on the form provided, within four (4) working days excluding Saturdays, Sundays, and Holidays, after his presentation.

Step 2. If the grievance is not satisfactorily settled at Step 1 of this procedure, an appeal therefrom may be taken by the Department Steward to the Employee Relations Manager or his designee. Such an appeal shall be valid only if the Steward so marks the grievance form within the time limit provided in Section "C" of this Article. The Employee Relations Manager, or his designee, will render a decision on a grievance so presented at Step 2 within three (3) working days, excluding Saturdays, Sundays and Holidays, after its presentation.

Step 3. If the grievance is not satisfactorily settled at Step 2 of this procedure, an appeal therefrom may be taken by the Chief Steward to the Personnel Director, or his designee. Such an appeal shall be valid only if the

Departmental Steward so marks the grievance form within the time limit provided in Section "C" of this Article.

The Personnel Director or his designee shall render a decision on a grievance so presented within three (3) working days, excluding Saturdays, Sundays and Holidays, after its presentation.

Step 4. If the grievance is not satisfactorily settled at Step 3, it may be submitted to arbitration upon the request of either the Hospital or the Union in accordance with Section "D" of this Article.

Section B. A grievance which affects a substantial number of employees and which the supervisor at Step 1 of this procedure lacks authority to settle, may initially be presented by the Chief Steward at Step 3.

Section C. 1. Any grievance not presented for disposition through the grievance procedure described in Section A, above, within five (5) working days, excluding Saturdays, Sundays and Holidays, after the occurrence of the condition giving rise to the grievance shall not thereafter be considered a grievance under this Agreement, unless a satisfactory reason is given in explanation of the failure to present the grievance within such time.

2. Should any appeal from the disposition of a grievance given at Step 1, 2, or 3 not be taken within three (3) working days, excluding Saturdays, Sundays and Holidays from the date of such decision, then the decision of such grievance shall be final and conclusive and shall not be reopened for discussion. Any disposition of a grievance accepted by the Union or from which no appeal has been taken shall be final and conclusive and binding upon all employees, the Hospital and the Union.

Section D. 1. Grievances as limited above, which are not settled at Step 3 of Section A may be referred to the American Arbitration Association for arbitration pursuant to its Rules.

2. The arbitrator shall have jurisdiction only over disputes arising out of grievances as to the interpretation or application of, or compliance with, the provisions of this Agreement.

3. The decision of the arbitrator shall be final and conclusive and binding upon all employees, the Hospital and the Union.

4. The arbitrator shall have no power to add to or subtract from or modify in any way any of the terms of this Agreement.

5. The administrative fees of the Association and the fee of the arbitrator shall be borne equally by the parties.

ADDENDUM B

THE GRIEVANCE HEARING

The Employee Relations Manager for General Hospital, Joe Thompson, received a written grievance form bypassing Steps 1 and 2 (Step 1 called for the employee and/or his union steward to present the case to the immediate supervisor; Step 2 provided for an appeal from the decision of the immediate supervisor to the department head) and submitting a Step 3 grievance in accordance with the collective bargaining agreement language which provided that "a grievance concerning a discharge or suspension *may* be presented initially at Step 3."

The employee, Harriet Hardluc, chose to submit her grievance to the third step of the grievance procedure. The meeting was called for 3 PM on September 2. It was held in the employee relations office of the Personnel Department. In attendance for the union were: the grievant, Ms. Hardluc, the union delegate (an elected employee from the grievant's department) and the union organizer (a paid employee of the union). Management was represented by the grievant's department head and first line supervisor. The grievance form containing the complete details as submitted by the grievant was read to all parties by Mr. Thompson, the Employee Relations Manager. It included the section of the collective bargaining agreement between the parties which in the employee's mind was violated by management: "Employee improperly terminated by management who did so arbitrarily and capriciously in direct violation of the contract's management rights clause."

The practice at General Hospital in all disciplinary actions was for management to present its case first at the third step hearing. The department head deferred to the first line supervisor, Mr. Gourmet, who made a detail presentation as follows:

> Ms. Hardluc has been employed by General Hospital for 18 years. All of her employment has been as a tray passer in the Food Service Department. This was a *second* termination for a poor attendance record. Her first termination was in July of 1976 which she appealed and the union finally took to arbitration in December of 1976. The arbitrator reduced the termination to a suspension *without back pay* and placed Ms. Hardluc on probation for a six month period during which she was clearly notified that her attendance record would be audited. The arbitrator in his decision enunciated the objective on the reduced punishment: The grievant's attendance must improve. She had been absent 26% of scheduled work days for a 13-month period preceding the discharge. If improvement was not demonstrated, the employee would be discharged.

Mr. Gourmet went on to discuss the second termination which is the subject of this third step hearing:

> On August 25, 1977, less than two months after the expiration of the probationary period (the six month period delineated by the arbitrator as a basis of reviewing the grievant's attendance record), the employee was terminated based on an absentee record of 30% from May 9, 1977, to August 19, 1977. Mr. Gourmet indicated to Mr. Thompson that he could no longer tolerate Ms. Hardluc's "abominable attendance record" which set a poor example for the rest of the department and transferred a burden to the remaining employees. He also stated that it was costly to permit such a poor attendance record since Ms. Hardluc's work responsibilities had to be handled through overtime which was paid at premium time as provided in the collective bargaining agreement. He took the final action of termination based upon the prior arbitration decision, and stated that such action was consonant with the handling of similar absentee problems in the Food Service Department. He then produced as evidence the employee's attendance record which reflected an absentee rate of 30% of scheduled work days for the three month period from May 9, 1977, through August 19, 1977.

The union organizer, a paid employee of the union representing the bargaining unit employees at General Hospital, Mr. Dewey Process, presented six arguments in support of Ms. Hardluc's grievance:

> 1. The record of 30% absences over the period from May through August 1977 was an inaccurate accounting. The employer should only have computed absenteeism statistics during the probationary period of January through July 1977, which was the period of measurement clearly indicated by the arbitrator. This would have resulted in an absentee record of $16\frac{2}{3}\%$.
> 2. Frequently a discharge for absenteeism is sustained where the grievant has very little seniority. It is rare that an employee with long service such as Ms. Hardluc is discharged, regardless of documented attendance records.
> 3. General Hospital has no formal program of absentee control. There was no published criteria or guidelines; thus, to discharge this employee is not justifiable.
> 4. In most cases of termination of long-term employees for absenteeism, proof of misconduct or poor work performance must be shown; otherwise, such termination is unusual based solely upon a poor absentee record.
> 5. Ms. Hardluc has a real health problem which the union medically documented in its presentation; thus, termination for a series of "involuntary" absences is unjust.
> 6. The employee has already been punished for her past absentee record and, therefore, her past record cannot serve as reason for the recent termination since this would constitute "double jeopardy."

Both presentations by the first line supervisor and the union organizer took approximately one hour. Mr. Thompson, the Employee Relations Manager, closed the hearing and informed the parties that the hospital's third step reply would be forthcoming within five working days as prescribed by the contract. That date would be September 9, 1977. The hospital's answer written on the grievance form follows:

> The hospital will reply to each of the six arguments submitted by the Union:
> 1. There is no rule which delimits the time of measurement of an employee's attendance record. The "staleness" of an absentee problem may be valid, but this is not the case. If the union's approach were correct, one might merely select the first three months of the probationary period where there was virtually no absenteeism at all. If such a rule were effected, a 20 year employee showing no absenteeism during the first 15 years and thereafter having an excessive record of absenteeism amounting to 30% of time during those last five years would have the rate of absenteeism computed over a 20 year period. It is much more realistic to select the last five year period of heavy absenteeism as a basis for computation.
> 2. Mr. Thompson cited several important arbitration decisions contrary to the union's contention and concluded that "there are indeed many additional cases wherein the discharges of long-term employees for absenteeism have been sustained."
> 3. The hospital maintains that the lack of a formal published program of absentee control is irrelevant in a case such as this one where the grievant was repeatedly warned about impending termination. She was personally put on notice of possible discharge if her absenteeism persisted. This was clearly indicated by the prior arbitrator's award.
> 4. Mr. Thompson's answer was similar to that regarding discharge of long-term employees, i.e., there are many cases which refute the Union's position.
> 5. Many past arbitration cases support the right of an employer to terminate an employee for poor attendance even if the reason for poor attendance is valid. The hospital cited several past arbitration summations on that issue:
> > a. Excessive absenteeism is one of the recognized grounds justifying discharge and it has been repeatedly held that where the circumstances warrant, the fact that an employee is incapacitated by forces beyond his or her control does not deprive the employer of the right to terminate employment;
> > b. The right to terminate employees for excessive absences even when they are due to illness is generally recognized by arbitrators;
> > c. Repeated absenteeism over a long period of time, even for valid reasons such as genuine illnesses, may make an employee of so little value if not an actual handicap to the institution as to justify a severance of the employment relationship.

6. It is true that the grievant paid for earlier rule infractions (warning notices, suspensions). This does not mean, however, that the grievant can act as though the infractions had never occurred in the first place. The logic of the union's argument would require erasing each instance from the employee's personnel file after discipline has been effected. The grievance file would then look as though there had never been any acts committed calling for discipline.

Mr. Thompson concluded management's answer at the third step with the following statement:

Management's decision to terminate Ms. Hardluc for poor attendance is hereby upheld.

The union wisely did not appeal management's third step denial of the grievance to arbitration.

ADDENDUM C

FINANCIAL AND ADMINISTRATIVE PRACTICES
OF ARBITRATORS*

A majority of arbitrators have raised their fees only once or not at all in the last five years, about one third of arbitrators reduce their fees under certain circumstances, and more than half of arbitrators charge fees for hearing cancellations. These were some conclusions drawn from a survey of arbitrators conducted by two Loyola University professors.

The survey—conducted by Donald J. Petersen, professor of management, and Julius Rezler, emeritus professor of economics—explored the financial and administrative practices of 97 arbitrators who completed three-page questionnaires. Those responding constitute 49 percent of a total of 198 arbitrators who were asked to participate.

In analyzing the data, the authors differentiate between members of the National Academy of Arbitrators and nonmembers and between lawyers and nonlawyers. Of those responding to the survey, 44, or 45 percent, are NAA members, and 51, or 53 percent, are lawyers.

The authors also found that 32 percent of the respondents are engaged in full-time arbitration practice, while 68 percent also are engaged in other occupations. The average age of the arbitrators is 57.9 years, and overall the sample is "heavily biased on the side of experienced arbitrators in accordance with the purpose of the study," the authors say.

One half of the arbitrators have raised their fees once in the last five years, the study found, while 15.6 percent have not raised fees, 27.1 percent have raised fees twice, and 7.3 percent have raised fees three or more times. NAA members raised their fees more often than nonmembers—almost half of the NAA respondents have raised their fees twice in five years (see Table 1).

The factor most frequently cited as influencing the size of per diem fees, accounting for 54.5 percent of responses, is a comparison with fees charged by arbitrators considered equal in experience and case load. Fee ranges reported by FMCS accounted for 21.6 percent of the answers, while fees charged by attorneys were mentioned in 9 percent of the response.

Asked whether the size of fees affected their arbitration caseload, 17.4 percent of the respondents replied yes and 80.3 percent answered no.

Thirty percent of the sample said that they reduce their fees under certain circumstances. In order of frequency, circumstances mentioned were the financial situation of the parties, whether or not costs are borne by

---

*Reprinted, with permission, from *Facts for Bargaining, Part 2 of What's New in Collective Bargaining Negotiations and Contracts,* No. 843, The Bureau of National Affairs, Inc. (September 22, 1977).

individual employees, lower fees fixed by law or by agencies, permanent umpireship, an unusual number of hearing days involved in a case, and a number of cases received from the same parties in a year *(see Table 2)*.

About half of the respondents charge for travel time when a minimum of one to four hours of traveling each way is required, the authors found. Ten percent do not charge for travel time.

The study shows that nearly one third of the sample consider fees overdue after one month, a third consider them overdue after two to three months, and one fifth do not have a policy on overdue fees. The most common action taken when fees are overdue is to write to the parties. About one fourth of the respondents feel that losing parties are slower to pay their fees.

Cancellation fees are regularly charged by 57.8 percent of the total, while 34 percent do not charge cancellation fees. The amount generally depends on how much notice is given, with one day's fee the most common charge. Most arbitrators charge a minimum of $25 plus expenses *(see Table 3)*.

Turning to the recordkeeping practices of arbitrators, the survey shows that a large majority retain copies of their awards permanently. Other types of records—notes, transcripts, briefs, exhibits, and correspondence—are kept for fewer than five years by a majority of respondents.

Table 1

Number of Times Arbitrators Have Raised Their Fees in the Past Five Years

Number of times respondents raised their fee in the last five years	Totals	Percent of Total	NAA Arbitrators			Non NAA Arbitrators		
			Lawyers	Non Lawyers	Percent of NAA Arbitrators	Lawyers	Non Lawyers	Percent of Non NAA Arbitrators
Zero	15	15.6	2	2	9.3	6	5	20.8
Once	48	50.0	9	6	34.9	12	21	62.3
Twice	26	27.1	10	10	46.5	2	4	11.3
Thrice	6	6.3	3	0	7.0	1	2	5.6
Five times	1	1.0	1	0	2.3	0	0	0.0
Totals	96 (a)	100.0%	25	18	100.0%	21	32	100.0%

(a) One respondent did not answer

Copyright © 1977 by The Bureau of National Affairs, Inc.

285

Table 2

Circumstances That May Cause Arbitrators to Reduce Their Per Diem

Circumstances	Totals	Percent of Total	NAA Arbitrators			Non NAA Arbitrators		
			Lawyers	Non Lawyers	Percent of NAA Arbitrators	Lawyers	Non Lawyers	Percent of Non NAA Arbitrators
The finnancial situation of one or both of the parties	14	25.4	6	3	26.5	8	2	23.8
Fee to be paid by an employee rather than by the parties	14	25.4	3	9	35.3	1	1	9.5
State or federal laws or agencies fix fee lower than arbitrator's regular fee	10	18.2	3	1	11.8	2	4	28.6
Permanent umpireship	5	9.1	0	1	2.8	1	3	19.0
Unusual number of hearing days involved in a case	5	9.1	2	2	11.8	0	1	4.8
Number of arbitration cases received from the same parties in a year	3	5.5	0	2	5.9	0	1	4.8
Others	4	7.3	2	0	5.9	1	1	9.5
Totals	55 (a)	100.0%	16	18	100.0%	8	13	100.0%

(a) does not add to 29, the total number of arbitrators who charge a variable fee, because more than one category could be selected.

Table 3

Notice Time Given By Parties For Cancellation and Fees Charged By Arbitrators

Notice Time Given for Cancellation	Fees Charged	Totals	Percent of Total
Less than 48 hours	One day's fee	7	11.3
Less than one week	One day's fee	23	37.1
One week to two weeks	½ day's fee One day's fee	5 7	8.1 11.3
15 days to three weeks	Varied between ¼ day's fee to one day's fee	4	6.4
One month	Varied between ½ day's fee to one day's fee	5	8.1
Any cancellation	Practices varied widely but most charged a minimum of $25 plus expenses. One respondent charged $50 and another $100 for any cancellation.	11	17.7
Totals		62 (a)	100.0%

(a) The total does not add to the number of arbitrators charging a cancellation fee (56) because it was possible to choose more than one category.

IX. THE PERSONNEL DIRECTOR: A PROFILE

In the bible of hospital administrators, MacEachern's giant tome, *Hospital Organization and Management,* the chapter on "Personnel Management in Hospitals" includes a statement about modern personnel management being one of the newest of the arts and sciences to be recognized by hospitals. The author comments that hospitals were slow to follow the lead of industry which had for a long time realized the necessity for good personnel relations and had built personnel management into a profession.[1] One observer pointed out that personnel management is a victim of administration. In conducting a limited survey of hospital board meetings, he was able to show that 40 percent of the time at these meetings was spent by the trustees talking about money, 20 percent about building improvement and equipment, 15 percent about medical staff problems, 10 percent about services, 10 percent about public relations and 5 percent about miscellaneous subjects *including personnel.*[2] Obviously the subject was not considered worthy of extended discussion!

Manpower management is one of the most important and complex responsibilities of the hospital administration. As previously discussed, 70 percent of the average hospital's and home's total budget is allocated for payroll or payroll-associated expenses. In spite of this staggering statistic, which points out the people-oriented nature of hospital administration, personnel administration in hospitals and related health care facilities has been too often the victim of the tendency on the part of some health care administrators to delegate responsibility to personnel directors with one hand and take it back with the other.

Modern health care institutions properly demand (or should demand) that the personnel department do more than recruit employees and maintain records. Hospitals and homes which do not have a professional broad-based program of recruitment, nor established well-written and well-communicated policies, and do not have sound wage and salary administration, have indeed failed in the elementary requirements for building a well-motivated and efficient work force.

The personnel director in a health care institution is an important and integral part of the administrative team which must direct its attention to arranging organizational conditions and methods of operation so that people can achieve *their* goals best by directing their efforts toward *organizational* objectives. This is a process primarily of creating opportunities, releasing potential, removing obstacles, encouraging growth and providing guidance.

Administrators should expect from their personnel directors the production of programs which afford employees the opportunity for continued self-development and the possibility of realizing their (the employees') own potentialities.

The influence and effectiveness of a health care institution's personnel department depends to a great extent on the support it receives from the director or administrator and from its board of trustees. It has been noted that if a health care institution simply appoints a personnel director and leaves him or her to sink or swim, the line supervisors are likely to ignore that individual and continue to make personnel decisions on their own. If, on the other hand, the administration makes it clear that the advice of the personnel department is to be taken seriously, its influence on day-to-day decisions will grow. Much depends also on the proficiency of the personnel staff in developing and "selling" sound personnel policies to the line supervisors and in giving helpful counsel without trying to usurp their authority.

Yoder pointed out that "Manpower management is not a new art . . . (it) is the procedure by which human resources are organized and directed in making the contribution to current social and individual goals." He amplified this by stating that "The primary job of manpower management is to develop effective programs for attaining these personal and social objectives through and in employment."[3] The activities of the personnel department are directed toward making line control of the human element stronger and more effective; in short, the personnel staff *recommends, cooperates* and *counsels* while line management actually *adopts* and *applies* the policies, techniques and procedures in its operations. It has been repeatedly affirmed that no matter how capable the members of the personnel staff may be, no matter how excellent the plan on which their activities are based, the personnel program cannot be successful unless the line organization is "doing a good personnel job at the workbench."[4]

Who Are the Personnel Directors?

The American Society for Hospital Personnel Administration conducted a survey and produced a profile on personnel directors in the hospital field in 1974. The following facts were ascertained:[5]

1. The average of all salaries reported was $16,778, an increase of 10 percent over the $15,282 average of 1972.

2. College graduates constitute 76 percent of the personnel directors, with 28 percent also holding master's degrees. In 1969, when an educational level question was included, a little over half of the directors were college graduates and only 17 percent had master's degrees.

3. Experience as a hospital personnel director averaged six years; while total experience as a personnel director averaged ten years. This is a drop of one year from the 1972 average experience of seven years as a hospital personnel director; total experience remained the same for both survey years.

The distribution of responses in 1974 was as follows: 78 percent were from directors of nongovernmental not-for-profit hospitals, 13 percent from directors of nonfederal governmental hospitals, 8 percent from investor-owned hospitals, and 1 percent from federal hospitals. Of the personnel directors responding, 25 percent were employed in hospitals of 201 to 300 beds; 24 percent in hospitals of 101 to 200 beds, 17 percent in hospitals of 301 to 400 beds; 15 percent in hospitals of 501 or more beds; 10 percent in hospitals of 401 to 500 beds; and 8 percent in the smallest hospitals, 100 beds or less.

Personnel directors in the Pacific region registered the highest percentage of replies, 23 percent, with the directors in the East South Central region registered the lowest, 2 percent. As in previous surveys, personnel directors of hospitals with 101 to 600 employees registered the largest response, 38 percent, and directors of hospitals with 601 to 1,200 employees registered the next largest response, 34 percent. Of the surveys received, 557 or 78 percent were from personnel directors of urban hospitals; 111 came from suburban hospitals, and 48 were from hospitals in rural areas. Of the 723 responses received, 672 included salary information.

From the data reported, the following composite of a hospital personnel director can be drawn:

> The hospital personnel director is a college-educated 41-year-old male who has been a hospital personnel director for 6 years and has a total of 10 years' experience as a personnel director. He is employed in a 301-to-400 bed hospital and directs between 601 to 1,200 employees. His hospital is located in a city, and he earns an annual salary of $16,778.

Women accounted for 196, or 27 percent, of the directors' responses this year. In past surveys, approximately 23 percent of the responses were from women. The average salary for a female personnel director in 1974 was $13,652 whereas the average salary for a male personnel director was

$18,057. However, only 43 percent of the females hold college degrees compared with 85 percent of the male personnel directors. Female personnel directors were employed mainly in smaller hospitals, those with fewer than 200 beds and hence fewer employees.

The ASHPA defined the personnel director's position as follows:

> Directs a personnel management program for a hospital or related health care facility. Duties include employment and placement functions, administering a formal wage and salary program which includes job evaluation and performance evaluation, administering employee relations services and formulating personnel policies. Employee training and education function, safety and labor relations activities may be included.[6]

In an interesting study of personnel directors, they were asked to distribute their working hours per week among typical personnel activities. This study conducted among a cross-section of industrial firms, produced the findings in Exhibit 1.[7] It is interesting to note the high percentage of time actually spent by personnel directors in making decisions for others. The study also indicated the percentage of time that personnel directors felt they should spend on each of the activities; in the main, they are satisfied with the time they spend—actually spend—on the various personnel activities. A most important element of this study was the discussion of the degree of commitment. *Personnel directors are almost as highly committed to their employing organization as they are to their occupation.* The occupation as a whole is only partially meaningful; therefore, personnel directors are only moderately committed to it. To make his work life meaningful, the personnel director must supplement his commitment to his occupation with some degree of organizational commitment.[8]

Some of the findings of this well-titled study *(An Occupation in Conflict)* are:[9]

1. Personnel directors as well as members of the two other personnel occupations studied (employment managers and vice presidents) are highly educated. Personnel people are no longer simply rejects from line management, but are highly trained specialists in personnel matters.

2. Personnel directors exhibit a high degree of intergenerational mobility at both the occupational and educational levels. In the main, personnel directors have come from fairly modest backgrounds and have been able to far outstrip their fathers.

3. There is some evidence that vice-presidents of personnel come from somewhat different family backgrounds than persons in the other two occupations (employment managers and personnel directors).

4. On activities performed by personnel directors, the only surprising

Exhibit 1

Activity	Actual %	Should %	Difference
Supervising subordinates	17%	14%	−3%
Planning personnel department activities	16%	20%	+4%
Representing company to outside organizations	5%	6%	+1%
Representing company to the union	10%	9%	−1%
Gathering information both inside and outside the organization	10%	6%	−4%
Providing information and advice for decision-making by others	17%	19%	+2%
Making decisions on personnel matters for other departments in the company	13%	11%	−2%
Involved in professional functions	4%	5%	+1%
Others	8%	10%	+2%

finding is the relatively large percentage of time (13 percent) spent on making decisions for other departments in the institution.

5. Personnel directors feel that they should be spending more time on planning personnel department activities, representing the institution in outside organizations, providing information and advice for decision-making by others and involving themselves in professional functions.

The personnel director in a health care facility often is the victim of two of the most important elements of his institution: the overriding predominance of the delivery of health care and financial restraints. In an attempt to deliver efficient and professional personnel administration to the organization, compromises must be made with these two major responsibilities of the organization. In the final analysis, programs, policies, procedures and decisions must at times be altered in order to maintain the delivery of care or similar compromises must be effected because of the financial limitations so prevalent in these institutions. Much of what he does is aimed at improving the lot of men at work. It is often done against the will of the workers and against the inertia and opposition of the administration he represents. Yet one keen observer of the profession points out that what the personnel director does is often more influential over who shall be engaged for work, what the employee will be paid for that effort and what his conditions of employment will be, than the desires of captains of industry themselves. Odiorne comments that to a large extent, they (personnel directors) have been the goad of the social conscience of industry, the representative of people in the dehumanized world of corporate endeavor.[10]

The successful personnel director in health care institutions, although faceless at times, seems to fit a mold. He or she is often extremely literate; the ability to "sell" programs is essential in the successful fulfillment of his or her responsibilities. In order to accomplish anything in an organization dominated by the line (medical staff), personnel executives must be more articulate and skilled in persuading others to accept their ideas than the line executives and medical staff with whom they deal. Often they are able to "command by default." Personnel problems may exist, and the line—because of a lack of time or interest—often does not address itself to these problems. Therefore, a dependence on the personnel executive grows. He must neutralize the negativeness of financial executives; he must work around the medical staff if it finds him an intruder. He must deal within the organizational structure which sets him at a disadvantage two or three levels below the director of the institution.

The industrial personnel director of yesterday and unfortunately today's hospital and home personnel director is often, at best, an employment manager. The requisition for personnel is forwarded to this computer-like service, the personnel department, whose prime responsibility (so the organization believes) is to place an ad, call an agency, conduct an interview and refer an applicant. It is therefore not unusual to find the "disadvantaged" organizational placement of the personnel department. In fact, a concomitant handicap is the inadequate quarters and poor location of the personnel department in most health care institutions.

The personnel director must fight for time and the ear of the top administrator. He often has no recourse to nor representative on the board of trustees. His programs are often measured short-sightedly in terms of immediate results rather than in the long-term benefits they may produce for the organization. Yet he occupies, or potentially can occupy, a position of prodigious responsibility affecting the life-style of the institution.

The personnel director who is to serve as an organizational leader in implementing an effective manpower management program must be more than an observer in the basic planning for staffing and "people" programs. By being an active member of the top administrative team, he should be participating in organizational planning—that is, projecting the organization into the future, evaluating present manpower and developing programs to improve skills and to maintain a stable yet dynamic organization. By doing this, he can be a focal resource individual. By maintaining adequate records, often computerized, he can provide surveys which indicate staffing patterns in similar organizations throughout the country and compare them with his present organization. He should have at his fingertips reports on the authorized table of organization for each department of the institution, turnover records, exit interview analyses, job descriptions and organization charts.

Personnel Ratios

Personnel ratio is defined as the number of personnel department employees for each one hundred (100) employees of an institution that are serviced. The Bureau of Labor Statistics reports[11] for the year 1975 the following personnel ratios (Ratio of personnel and labor relations workers per 100 total employees):

Construction	.21
Non-Durable Goods Manufacturer	.22
Finance, Insurance & Real Estate	.21
Local Government	.22
Federal Government	.73
State Government	4.63
Transportation, Communications and Public Utilities	.10

In a study conducted by the author in 1977 of large, nonprofit, voluntary hospitals in New York City, the following personnel ratios were established:

Number of Total Employees	Number of Personnel Department Employees	Personnel Ratio
7100	24	.34
6800	33	.49
6000	30.5	.51
5100	26	.51
4500	22	.49
4000	22.5	.56
3300	18	.55
2700	9.5	.35
2500	12	.48
2400	13	.54

Labor Relations vs. Personnel Administration

Collective bargaining introduces certain functions and procedures which were not found in the nonunion health care institution. The director of personnel in the unionized institution must now concentrate primarily on administration's dealings with the union. He or his subordinates must follow through on grievance cases filed by the union, represent the health care institution's cases at arbitration hearings, assemble data for contract negotiations and handle numerous other responsibilities which are born of the new collective bargaining relationship. Once the union enters the health care institution as a legitimate representative of the employees, a major responsibility of the personnel department is dealing with the elected agent of the employees in interpreting the terms of the collective bargaining agreement. It is imperative that the primary responsibility for advice on labor-management relations be delegated to the personnel executive. This responsibility includes a minimization of internal conflict without sacrificing financial responsibility and control, or limiting the efficiency of delivering sound patient care. Labor relations activities in health care institutions can be viewed as having a primarily organizational maintenance function.[12]

The dilemma here is that often characteristics associated with the successful personnel director are at variance with those of the successful labor relations administrator. The latter is often put in an adversary position with the unionized employees. He must be a hard negotiator, often circumscribed in his ability to compromise by financial restraints and the need to protect management rights. He has been likened to a quarterback on a professional football team whose coach sends in the signals, and who must execute the plays (some of which he may disagree with). He must turn down some employee requests. He is often "Mr. Hardnose." Conversely, the successful personnel director is a friend of the employees. He represents the men to management and management to the men. He spends most of his time devising and implementing programs which will benefit the rank and file as well as the institution. When both these functions are delegated to one individual, requirements for the successful fulfillment of that role are geometrically increased.

In order to operate within the context of a unionized situation, the personnel director must have optimum authority and maximum influence. Eby lists the following major requirements of a sound labor relations program and of a successful labor relations executive:[13]

1. Top management must determine where the field of industrial relations fits into the administrative picture. Does it line up with some of the more important responsibilities?

2. Administration must decide on the degree and extent of union recognition.

3. Administration must vest in its director of personnel adequate authority for him to carry out the responsibilities of his post. Thereafter, he

must prepare and guide through to acceptance by administration the basic policies necessary to implement his responsibilities.·

4. The director of personnel must make certain that all levels of administration understand and agree with the institution's basic policy in labor relations and the way it will be administered in day-to-day contacts with all levels of union representatives.

5. The director of personnel should patiently, but determinedly, work to remove roadblocks to labor/management understanding and co-operation.

6. The personnel director is responsible for making sure that advance preparation, planning and assembling of facts have been accomplished before contract negotiations begin.

7. After a settlement, there exists the obligation to fully indoctrinate all levels of supervision on every detail of the settlement.

8. The director of personnel should develop for his institution a code of ethics and a management philosophy for personnel administration in general, and labor relations in particular, that will meet the test of being firm but fair, tough but tender, and hard but human.

It is obvious from this list that the functions of labor relations executives in health care institutions must be placed at an extremely high level of the organization. In fact, those institutions in the health care field that have labor contracts invest more authority in their personnel director and pay higher salaries than the nonunionized institutions.

Conclusions

One of the more important responsibilities of the health care institutions is for personnel administration. *People* render care to the sick and the needy. Hospitals and homes are in the business not of manufacturing things, but of rendering services. Service industries are far more dependent than others upon employee morale and commitment. Employees in such institutions are constantly facing the public. More often than not, patients refer to the presence or lack of "tender, loving care." Institutions which provide medical care will be criticized more for the *attitudes* of their personnel than for the *quality* of the care. It is difficult to accept, but nevertheless a valid observation, that patients and visitors are more impressed and concerned with the attentiveness, empathy and responsiveness of the health care worker than with the financial aspects of their exposure to an institution. The highly sophisticated and complex environments now operative in health care institutions in our society mandate that individuals responsible for the personnel function no longer communicate and implement by the seat of their pants. They must:

1. Develop a job evaluation program.
2. Write a policy manual.
3. Write an employee handbook.
4. Develop and effect an orientation and induction program.
5. Develop, implement and review performance evaluation programs.
6. Embark upon a management development program.
7. Administer the grievance procedure.
8. Initiate new and constructive employee relations programs.
9. Continuously survey the needs of their organization.
10. Develop a staff of competent associates and assistants.
11. Maintain an effective level of productivity in the organization.
12. Maintain an organizational life-style which produces high employee morale and satisfaction.
13. Represent the men to management and management to the men.
14. Spearhead the organization's position vis-à-vis unions.

More often than not, as staff administrators, they must make line administration believe that they (the line administrators) make the decisions while still maintaining their (the personnel directors') power. It is not easy for line managers and chairmen of departments to take orders from the personnel director. Personnel administration focuses the attention of administrators and medical men upon the social and psychological side of the enterprise. It does this by giving sound advice to both these segments of the institution, *not by giving orders.*

Dale Yoder, who has done more for codifying the profession than any other individual, states that "Manpower management must give more attention to the satisfaction of fundamental, psychological and social needs of employees if it is to perform its function with greatest effectiveness."[14]

Notes

1. Malcolm T. MacEachern, *Hospital Organization and Management* (Chicago: Physicans Record Company, 1957) , p. 961.
2. William R. Christopher Management Enterprises, St. Louis, Missouri.
3. Dale Yoder, *Personnel Principles and Practices* (Englewood Cliffs, N.J.: Prentice-Hall, Inc., 1956), p. 1.
4. "How to Establish and Maintain a Personnel Department," No. 4 (New York: American Management Association, 1944), *passim.*
5. *American Society for Hospital Personnel Administration 1974 Profile: Hospital Personnel Director* (Chicago, August, 1974).
6. *Idem.*

7. George Ritzger and Harrison M. Trice, *An Occupation in Conflict: A Study of the Personnel Manager* (Ithaca, N.Y.: New York State School of Industrial and Labor Relations, Cornell University, 1969), p. 19.

8. *Ibid.*, p. 45.

9. *Ibid.*, pp. 79-80.

10. George S. Odiorne, *Personnel Policies: Issues and Practices* (Columbus, O.: Charles E. Merrill Books, Inc., 1963), pp. 52-3.

11. "Occupational Employment Patterns for 1960 and 1975," *Bureau of Labor Statistics Bulletin No. 1595*, Bureau of Labor Statistics, 1968.

12. Norman Metzger and Dennis D. Pointer, *Labor-Management Relations in the Health Services Industry* (Washington, D.C.: Science and Health Publications, Inc., 1972), p. 199.

13. Herbert O. Eby, *A Business-Like Approach to Labor Relations: The Personnel Function: A Progress Report*, No. 54 (New York: American Management Association, 1958), pp. 61-9.

14. Yoder, *op. cit.*, p. 9.